Reflections on Medicine and Humanity

REFLECTIONS ON MEDICINE AND HUMANITY

Prose, Poetry, and Art - By MAVEN Project Physician Volunteers

Published by: MAVEN Project PO Box 156781
San Francisco, California 94115
https://www.mavenproject.org/

Editors: Barbara Loeb, MD & LoAn Nguyen, MD
Cover Art and Photography Editor: David C. Hurwitz, MD

Printed in the United States of America

ISBN 979-8-9869154-0-1

Reflections on Medicine and Humanity

Prose, Poetry, and Art

MAVEN Project
Physician Volunteers

Edited by: Barbara Loeb, MD & LoAn Nguyen, MD

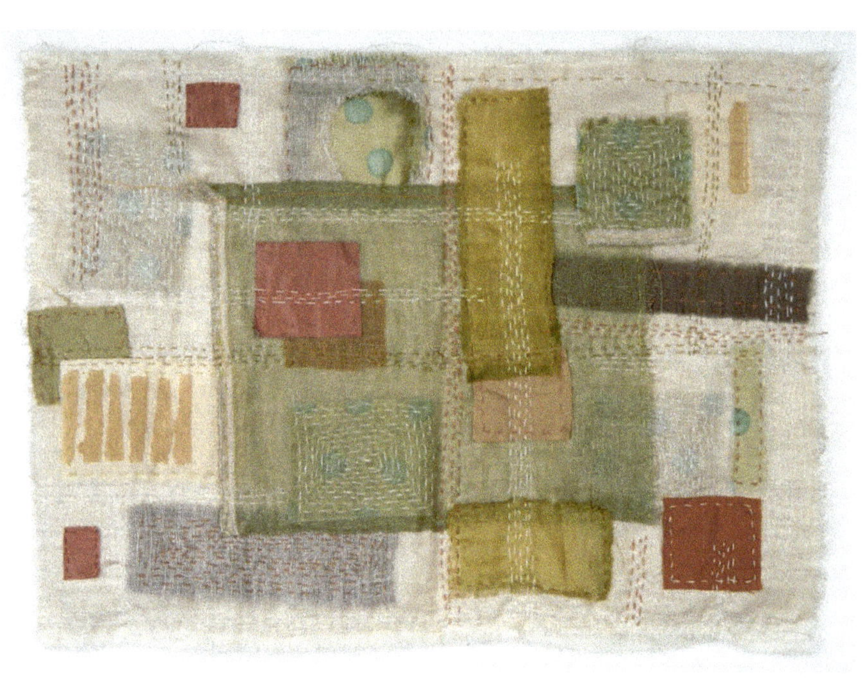

Summer Steps - boro textile by Jeanne Reisman, MD

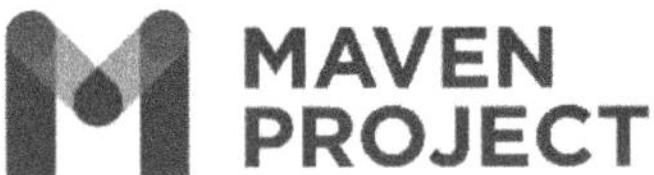

MAVEN Project is a national nonprofit organization working to address the social, racial, and economic inequities in health care. MAVEN Project connects frontline providers with a network of expert physician volunteers via telehealth for peer-to-peer consultations, medical education, and 1:1 mentoring.

MAVEN Project partners exclusively with community health centers and free and charitable clinics to support patients who often face numerous barriers to specialty care, including long wait times, travel, and out-of-pocket costs. Additionally, frontline providers are supported, and the knowledge they gain with each consultation and education session is applied to future patients.

MAVEN Project's corps of volunteers draws upon years of clinical experience and earned wisdom to help frontline providers in partner clinics. Volunteers are dedicated to the organization's mission and give generously of their time and talents.

MAVEN Project

Table of Contents

Table of Images

Out of Isolation - Lake Havasu - photograph
Barbara Loeb, MD

Reaching and Hope - marble
Kenneth Elconin, MD

Mist Trail at Yosemite - photograph
Cynthia A. Point, MD

Trees - watercolor
Jan Herr, MD

Sphinx #1 - marble
Kenneth Elconin, MD

Preface

A year and a half ago, as we were preparing for a presentation on communication skills, the two of us began sharing stories about our patient care experiences over our combined more than sixty years of practice. We reflected on how often we were so busy in our constant daily responsibilities that we did not fully recognize the wisdom that our patients imparted to us, nor how often their stories shaped us as healers. With this epiphany, we recognized a unique opportunity to form a narrative writing group among MAVEN Project physician volunteers. The participants wrote stories and poetry derived from their careers and personal lives which served as a way of reflecting and connecting. The group was named "Narrative and Humanity", and its efforts became the inspiration for this book.

The COVID-19 pandemic coincided with the retirements of many MAVEN Project physician volunteers. This global emergency, coupled with facing the implications of our professional transitions, became the impetus for pausing and recognizing the fullness of our clinical years and telling individual stories. In addition to being a series of reflections, the book is a celebration of the authors and artists' personal lives.

The diverse backgrounds, experiences, and perspectives of the "Narratives and Humanity" collective provided an excellent milieu for writing, and listening. Members wrote in response to monthly themes; both prose and poetry flowed from the contributors during each Zoom session. After eight months, this community of writers had produced an archive of thoughtful pieces worthy of sharing, prompting the creation of this book. As we put the compendium together, we identified the creative talents among the physician volunteers extended beyond the written words. They contributed photography and images of watercolor paintings, charcoal drawings, ceramics, marble sculptures, textiles, and wood carvings. The artistry of these visual additions beautifully complemented the prose and poetry.

As you read each piece and take in the artwork, we hope you gain a deeper sense of humanity in the hearts of the authors and artists and find your own creative expression.

Barbara Loeb, MD & LoAn Nguyen, MD
Editors

Introduction

This book is arranged in five chapters. The written pieces and artworks are grouped into themes which metaphorically mark phases of the contributors' careers and life journeys.

Chapter One – *Giving & Receiving:* Presents the gratitude of giving and receiving gifts from our surroundings, experiences, and relationships, both professionally and personally.

Chapter Two – *Early Journeys*: Visits vivid memories and events from childhood and young adulthood, poignant recollections that provide glimpses into how our early experiences help shape our futures.

Chapter Three - *What Patients Teach Us:* Highlights stories about patient experiences, illustrating not only what the physicians learn about patients, but also what they learn from their patients and in the process about themselves. This provides a rich territory filled with lessons to share. As readers look through the author's eyes, the words will resonate for both the givers and receivers of care.

Chapter Four – *Pandemic Pause*: Presents a juxtaposition of pieces produced during the COVID-19 pandemic. The writings and artworks capture the impact of this challenging time, when many paused and asked important questions about life and priorities.

Chapter Five – *Humanity & Resilience*: Provides a collection of personal writings and images that focus on the power to endure adversity and embrace compassion.

CHAPTER ONE
Giving & Receiving

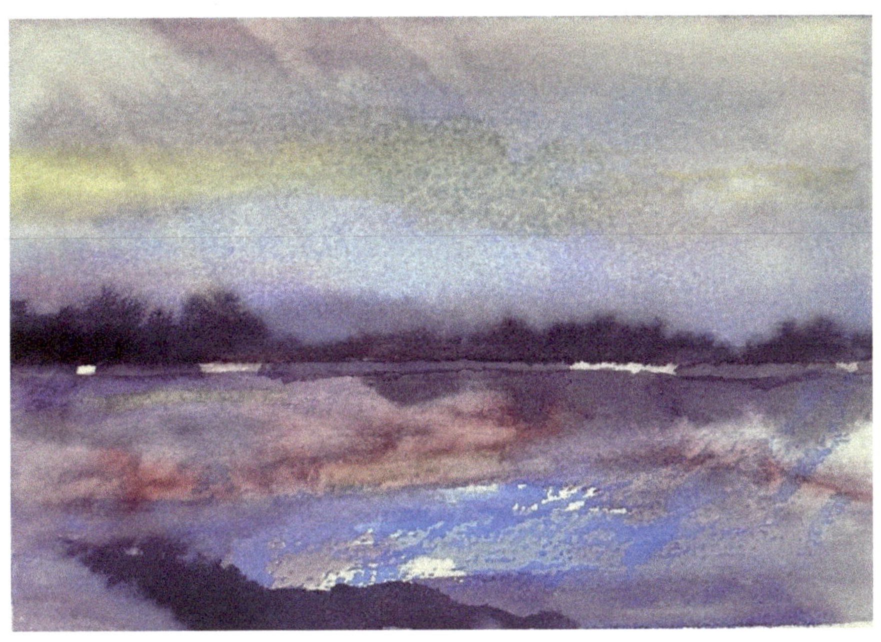

Mauve Storm - watercolor by Jan L. Herr, MD

Shoes

By Barbara Loeb, MD

If you could walk
   a mile in my shoes
      you might not pause
    until your feet blister

you might not notice
   the rhythm of your heels
      striking the sidewalk
   or feel the wind lifting your hair

you might not be startled
   by ambulance screeches
      rushing to save lives
    or notice a double rainbow
     its multicolored arcs
    illuminating the sky.

If you were in my shoes
   you might miss your heart is aching
    from losses you've tried hard to forget
        or think you're unscathed
      by unkind words spoken
       even your own.

  Unaware, your eyes might avoid
      connecting with those
     of a tattered soul sitting alone
       on the sidewalk

you might not try to imagine
        what it would be like
                to be in their shoes

                not realizing that you
                        could be that stranger
                                that their journey
                                is your journey.
        Fearful, you might fail
                to extend your hand
                        or your heart–

If you could walk
        a mile in my shoes
                you might find
                your feet no longer lift
                until you've stopped
                to face that stranger

                not knowing what to do
                        you lower your body
                                sit patiently by their side

                        until the line between you blurs
                and two pairs become one.

The Hospital Police Officer Who Saved the Day

By Charles E. Schwartz, MD

My beeper went off that afternoon.

It was the head nurse on a medical floor.

"We have a problem. Can you come right up?"

Off the elevator, I was met by a crowd congregated around the nursing station – nurses and aides. I recognized a hospital administrator, the nursing supervisor, and the director of Hospital Police. I took a minute to carefully scan the group, but after looking around, none of his doctors were to be found.

All eyes were on me.

The story unfolded, as the nurses spoke:

"Ray, a twenty-four-year-old man slowly dying from AIDS, had finally succumbed midday."

I knew Ray. I had been seeing him periodically since his admission, as a consultant to his medical team.

The nurse making rounds had found Ray unresponsive, pulseless, and apneic. He was a "no code," so she had drawn the curtain, and quietly left the room and closed the door.

The head nurse paged the house staff, while Ray's roommate had been quickly moved to another room. His resident "pronounced" Ray dead; the intern called Ray's mother, Maria, who came right away, and was in the room.

Then, as per hospital protocol, the nurses wrapped and covered Ray, but when they started to bring in the morgue stretcher, Maria refused. Ray couldn't be moved until his younger sister, Angela, came from high school, as she had done every day during his hospitalization.

Well over an hour had passed since Ray's death when Angela arrived.

She exited the elevator and came onto the unit, but no one thought to speak with her to in any way prepare her, and she went right in. She screamed when she saw Ray lying there, wrapped up like a mummy, in the middle of an otherwise empty room. She ran to him and flung herself onto his bed, holding him tightly, and began to sob, as she took the chair near her mother.

When a nurse came in a few minutes later and told her that they had to take Ray to the morgue, Angela cried out and ran to his bed. Once again, she lay down next to him clinging to his body, keening.

Unable to get her to disengage, the nurse left and spoke with the nursing supervisor, who had paged me.

A hush fell over the group.

All eyes turned to me. I was supposed to fix this.

The first thing that came to my mind: where were Ray's doctors? Though livid, I would have to come back to that later.

I walked past the empty gurney to Ray's room and knocked on the closed door.

A hospital police officer, who had been stationed just inside the room, opened the door just enough to let me in.

I entered the room, and the officer closed the door behind me.

Ray lay in his hospital bed in the center of the almost empty room. He was wrapped in a white shroud like a mummy, arms folded tightly over his chest, legs bound together. Only his face was uncovered, ringed by the folds of the shroud, poised ready to fully enclose him.

Angela lay beside him, holding him tightly, quietly sobbing, intermittently rocking, and calling his name, while Maria sat in a chair against the far wall, her gaze locked on the bed.

I had no idea what to do.

I looked to Maria, trying to catch her attention, hoping for her help, but she sat silently, motionless, gazing straight ahead at her children.

"Hello Angela. I'm Dr. Schwartz," I began.

...Silence.

"I'm one of the doctors caring for your brother, and I am so sorry that Ray died. The doctors and nurses have told me how close you two are." (Hoping that would set the right tone.)

Angela's sobbing grew louder.

"Ray is not dead," she said flatly, without even looking up at me.

"Angela, I wish he wasn't dead." (Telling myself that she was just being metaphoric)

"Ray is not dead," she said insistently, again and again, her face pressed against his body, her sobs becoming wailing.

"Angela, this is so hard. I know how close you two are, and how much you wish he wasn't dead." (Hoping to find some common ground.)

She said nothing, tightening her grip on Ray, as I stood silently.

I had no idea what to do next.

Then there was a loud knock at the door, and an administrator strode in, imperious. In a commanding tone edged with irritation, she said:

"It has been almost two hours, and it is hospital policy - we have to remove the body so that we can clean this room and get it ready for another patient."

I became enraged. Angela had only gotten to the hospital a few minutes before, and the staff had summoned me to the unit asking me to help, but now they weren't even giving me a chance to try.

"No, we don't," I barked.

With a shocked expression on her face the supervisor backed out of the room and closed the door. (I was a little shocked myself.)

Then I glanced over at Angela.

The sobbing had stopped, and she had loosened her hold on Ray, and had a slight smile on her face. Angela now felt that I was on her side. The tension in the room had been broken.

"You haven't had a chance to really say goodbye yet," I told her, *"and I want you to have a few minutes. THEY, can wait."*

"Thank you," Angela responded.

I took a seat opposite Maria, as we watched brother and sister.

After a few minutes, and after I gently repeated our shared "wish" that Ray had not died, Angela loosened her hold, and began to get up from the bed.

The officer also rose, opened the door, and began to wheel in the morgue stretcher.

It looked like a streamlined aluminum sarcophagus on wheels, and as he moved it towards the bed, Angela stiffened, lay back down, and grabbed her brother.

"If you cover his face and you put him in there, Ray won't be able to breathe," Angela said, with a far-away sound in her voice. The officer backed away and returned to his seat by the door.

I sighed. The tension mounted again, as the minutes passed.

What could I say? Did we really have to cover his face? Could we take him to the morgue this way? Maybe Ray didn't need to be fully shrouded, and encased in that sarcophagus? But then what was going to happen when Ray got to the morgue, since Angela didn't seem to believe that he was dead?

This was bad. I looked at Maria, but she remained silent. I turned to the officer with a questioning, plaintive look on my face, but he just shook his head, very slightly, from side to side. What had I expected? He didn't know what to do either.

Minutes passed.

Then he got up and walked slowly toward Angela, speaking softly and gently.

"Angela, we need to move Ray to the stretcher, and we need to cover him. In a few minutes, we will be taking him out of this room, down the hall, and into the elevator. Other people use that elevator too, and we don't want them staring. It just wouldn't be right. Ray needs his privacy."

She considered this for a minute, then nodded, and loosened her grip.

He rolled the stretcher alongside the bed, lifted off the shroud cover, and gently placed it on the floor.

"Angela, I need you to help me with this," he continued softly.

Ray was so terribly thin and wasted, after his long battle with AIDS.

The officer picked up the end of the sheet under Ray's head, looking toward Angela.

I held my breath, until she nodded, got up, and walked to the foot of Ray's bed and grasped the sheet.

"One, two, three," he said, and they both pulled Ray onto the gurney.

He stepped back, moved to one end of the cover, and motioned to Angela, who went to the other end. They lifted the shroud, gently setting it down, covering Ray.

The officer went to the door, opened it, and nodded. An aide entered.

"Angela, he will guide the stretcher, and I'll walk with you and your mother, right behind Ray. We will go with him into the elevator, and down to the morgue. I want you to make sure that they treat your brother with respect."

He walked over to Maria, offered her his hand, and helped her to her feet. As the aide began to push the stretcher, Maria followed, and holding Angela's hand, she and the officer followed closely behind. I watched in amazement, as they proceeded down the hall, and into the elevator...

Several hours later, I found the officer manning the hospital entrance and asked him what had happened. He said that the trip to the morgue had been uneventful.

"After Angela got Ray settled, I took Maria and Angela to the coffee shop, for a cup of coffee. We talked for a few minutes, and they were fine. I gave them my condolences, and I saw them to the door."

I looked at him in awe.

"You deserve a medal, you know." He just smiled, walking back to his post.

The next day I wrote a letter to the Director of Hospital Police, describing what had happened, urging him to give the officer a commendation.

That was almost thirty years ago, now. No one gave much thought to multidisciplinary health care "teams." We did not see past doctors, and surely no further than nurses.

But that day my eyes were opened by the wisdom and gentle skill of this officer, who saved the day.

What I learned from this officer; I will never forget.

And I try not to forget my humility.

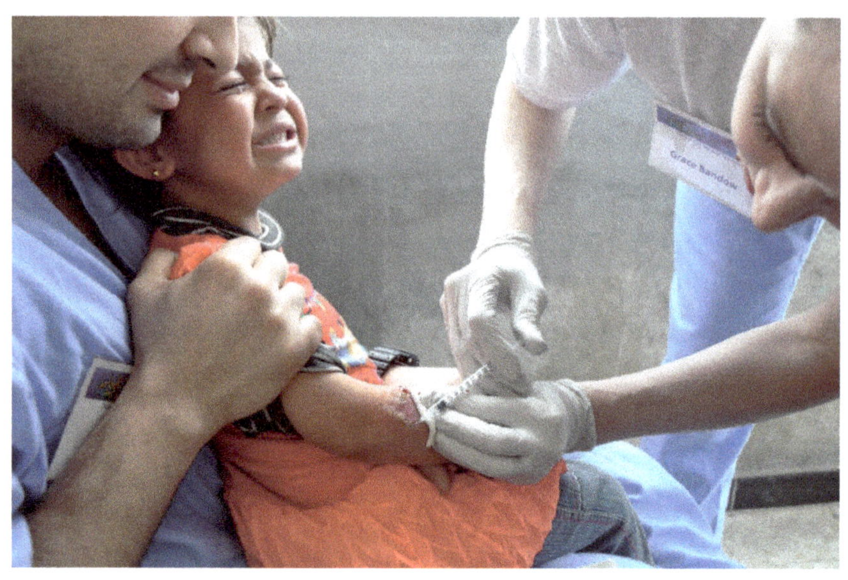

Treating Cutaneous Leishmaniasis - photograph of Grace D. Bandow, MD

What does a Dermatologist do in a Syrian Refugee Camp?

By Grace D. Bandow, MD

This is what we heard several times as we prepared for our medical mission to Jordan. After all, these people are suffering from such traumas as rape, torture, limb loss, gunshots, eviction; they are suffering the tragedy that is genocide. They have fled to save their lives, leaving behind their sons, homes, jobs, and schools. They need food, clean water, and obstetric care, certainly not treatment for their *acne.* What exactly *were* we going to do there?

We were two busy dermatologists, working hard, comfortable in our communities. Over the last three years, we watched as the Syrian crisis unfolded from a minor uprising to a seemingly endless decimation of an entire country. It was another news story, covered in brief, digestible sound bites on the evening news, wedged between updates on the Affordable Care Act and the birth of a royal baby. When we received an email request from a Syrian American doctor, who leads medical missions, we felt compelled to answer. He was asking for help, of any kind. We were searching for a fresh perspective, of any kind.

Living in poverty can create big medical problems. Living in close, dirty quarters transforms minor diseases left untreated into major problems. Without relief, nuisances multiply, eventuating in real misery.

We anticipated scabies, lice, and impetigo of crowded living. It never occurred to us to prioritize Vaseline petroleum jelly as an item of high importance when we packed our supplies for the Syrian refugee camps. After all, it was heavy stuff, and the airlines were counting pounds.

Then we met a man in Deir Alla. He stood in line quietly, waiting with dozens of others at dusk, for an opportunity to talk to the American doctors. When he got his turn, he offered us the bottom of his feet and showed us their deep, painful cracks. His feet were worn out from traveling hundreds of miles on hot sandy soil in rubber sandals. He told us that if he could fix his feet, maybe he could find a job to support his children. He had been a civil engineer in Syria. He used to have a home. He used to have dignity and freedom. Now, he is confined to a tent, waiting. He asked us for Vaseline.

In Amman, we met a twelve-year-old girl with a universally fatal blistering skin disease. She was malnourished because her mouth was full of blisters, making it impossible for her to chew solid food. She smelled bad because her wounds were infected, and her bath was available only once a month with a hose and cup. She sat silently in front of us, wrapped from her neck to her toes in soiled gauze dressings, tears slowly dripping down one side of her pale face as her mother told us their story. In Syria, her daughter had good care and a daily regimen that allowed her to function. When they arrived in Jordan, all the hospitals rejected her. Her husband is missing. Five of her brothers are dead. With her four children, she left to save their lives. She needed something as simple as a tub and salt to make a proper bath for her daughter. She needed basic supplies like gauze to wrap her chronic wounds. She needed Vaseline to put under the gauze.

We met a man with dry broad scars across his arms. He explained that after moving to the refugee camp, his tent was caught on fire. His arms were burned when he tried, unsuccessfully, to pull his two-year-old son from the flames. He wanted to tell us his story. And he did. We listened in horror as he explained why he left his country to live on a dirt floor, in a tent that burned and took his child. He smiled as he spoke, showing us his skin over and over, showing us that it was dry and that the dry parts itched. We nodded and listened and agreed, realizing he too needed something as simple as Vaseline.

These stories continued for hours every day. Days blended together and quickly became a week. Hundreds of patients lined up to show us their skin, but really to tell us their stories. After all, they didn't need treatment for their acne and eczema as much as they needed to know that someone cared that they existed. A woman whose children were forced to witness the gang rape of their father before he was thrown off their balcony, already knows she will deal with this for the rest of her life. What she doesn't know is whether the world cares. This is why she stood in line.

The tragedy in Syria is a human tragedy. It is the tragedy of war, of ruthless dictators, of brutal force, of genocide against an entire country.

As doctors, we were able to treat a few specific problems in several hundred people. What a daunting task in the face of nine million refugees, with nine million stories. These are people who survive through the generosity of the international community. They survive through the human will to live and by the simple ability to wait.

As medical students, interns, and residents, we are trained to assess situations, move quickly, triage accurately, and to identify and respond to problems, both acute and chronic. We are trained to make use of available resources and to improvise when they are scarce. Leaving our own thriving practices to work in a crowded, dusty refugee camp in another part of the world, we were reminded that sometimes simple measures, like compassion and listening are what is most vital to a human being; and that sometimes basic, inexpensive remedies, like Vaseline, are sufficient treatment for a medical problem.

Since returning, their stories continue to haunt our daily lives. We can see their faces and we can hear their voices, always repeating the same simple request. "Please, we want to go back to our homes; we want our children to go to school; we want you to share our story."

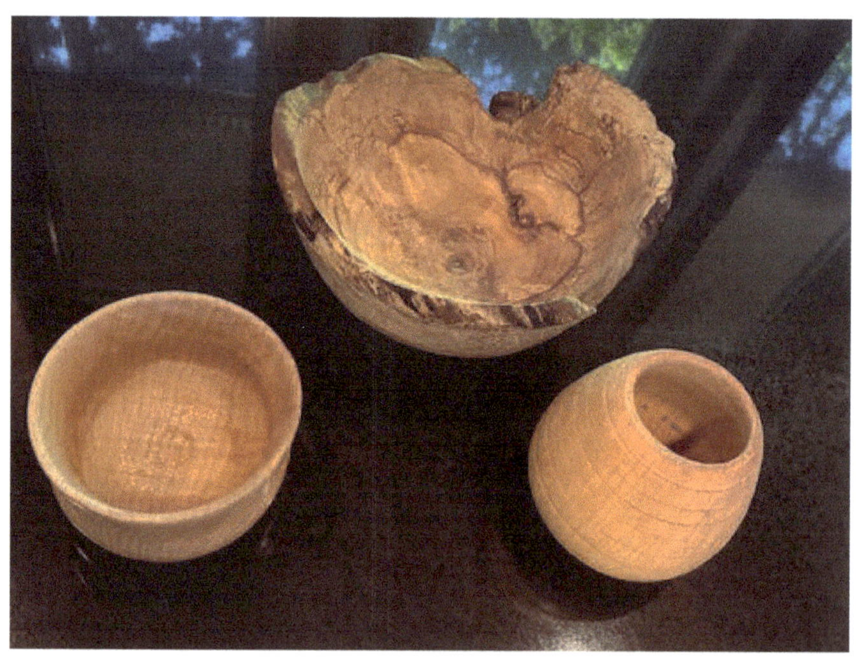

Three Bowls on Black - bigleaf maple by Tom E. Norris, MD

Gratitude

By Michael E. Day, MD

Not all gifts are made of material things. A simple word of thanks can be construed as a gift, and at times it can mean as much or more than any other gift. This story is about a "gift" given to me by a patient some years ago.

Earl was a patient who I saw regularly and rather frequently until the time that I retired from full-time practice in 2013. I could usually tell when he had made his appearance in my office by the laughter coming down the hallway as Earl was telling my medical assistants, in his loud voice, one of his numerous corny jokes. He always seemed to have a truckload of new jokes to tell me and others in the office, so I had to brace myself when I went in the exam room with him. In fact, I came to be able to tell how bad Earl was feeling just by the number of jokes that he told me, as well as the vigor with which he told them. If he was somber and not telling jokes, you knew he was in bad shape!

Earl was also a musician and a trumpet player who composed a lot of his own music. Almost every visit consisted of time reviewing his progress on his latest composition. Consequently, an office visit with Earl typically took a little longer than most. However, I was generally happy to take this extra time with him, in particular because of how Earl was so enthusiastic about leaving a legacy of his music to his granddaughter and to others.

Unfortunately, he had a number of medical problems. Earl suffered from extreme obesity among other things. All of my efforts through the years to get him to significantly lose and sustain weight loss were unsuccessful. He had a severe case of chronic leg edema, probably at least partly the result of his obesity. He also suffered from hypertension that was difficult to control, and high cholesterol. He had an enlarged heart as the result of all these problems, which usually means a weak heart. Earl had multiple risk factors for heart disease. He was, as we sometimes say, a "heart attack waiting to happen."

So, it was no surprise to me when one morning Earl presented to my office complaining of shortness of breath that had increased over the past day, increasing weakness, and some pressure in his chest. He did not have any jokes for me that day and was obviously worried and in physical distress.

It did not take a great diagnostician to recognize that he may be having a heart attack. It did not take exceptionally fine hearing for me to recognize the crackles in the bases of his lungs, signifying that his heart was weak and could be failing. It did not take great decision making to whisk him over to the emergency room by ambulance and notify a cardiologist of his condition. This was not a tough call. I just did what I would expect myself and other physicians to do. Dr. House was not needed for consultation! I would never be able to impress my colleagues at a medical convention about my great medical exploits in this case!

Fortunately, Earl did well and recovered rather uneventfully from his heart attack. He was stabilized on medication and got back to his usual bubbly and joking self. I was, of course, happy for him, but I was unprepared for the degree of gratitude that Earl showered on me. He was convinced that I had saved his life, and vociferously thanked me for this.

Perhaps a year later I had a retirement party thrown for me by my coworkers at about the time that I retired from full-time practice. Many of my longtime patients had been invited and attended this gathering, as well as my coworkers, many doctors, and other people who I had worked with through the years. It was a very emotionally touching event for me.

As I was circulating through the crowd that evening, trying to greet as many people as possible, I overheard Earl's booming voice several times telling someone that I was the doctor who saved his life. I could not have asked for any more beautiful background music! I was the one who was grateful to Earl for his compliments and trust in me.

Remembering Martha

By Carrie A. Horwitch, MD

The casserole was ready to be taken out of the oven. I reached into the drawer and pulled out a handmade hot pad. It was a gift from Martha G.

Mrs. G was one of my first patients during my internal medicine residency. Our medical clinic was designed to take care of the underserved. We took patients with Medicare, Medicaid, and those without insurance. Martha was in her sixties when I met her. She had high blood pressure and borderline diabetes. Over time, she also developed congestive heart failure symptoms. She always came to clinic dressed conservatively, with her hair carefully coiffed. She was quiet and would always calmly answer my long list of medical questions. "How are you feeling today?" "Are you taking your medications?" "Are you having any chest pain or shortness of breath?" She would put up with my complete physical examination as well.

I saw her several times over the three years of my residency training. Sometime in my last year of training Mrs. G. gave me a poem she had written. I was surprised. I had no idea that she wrote poetry. Knowing that poetry is often an intimate personal expression, I was pleased that she felt comfortable enough to share it with me.

A Visit to See the Doctor by Martha G.

Well, I went to see the Doctor…
It was just a routine check:
The Doctor said, you take these pills,
And in 2 weeks, I'll see you back.

So I stepped up to the window
To place my ID card up there.
Then I found a place to be seated,
And just sit down without a care!

Soon, someone will weigh you in
And take all your vitals, too
Now, you must not gain more weight
Whatever it is, that you do:
The nurse will probably ask you then
If you need a blood test
While you're trying hard to relax,
Oh, you're doing your very best

Then she says, you come with me…
Into this little lab room!
Put your arm upon this board…
And I'll stick you real soon!

You may go back and be seated now
And just wait there for a spell
And when the Doctor gets ready for you
She will see if you are well!

Down the Hall then we go…
And we turn to the right:
And set there a little while
With my heart filled with fright!

But now, the Doctor comes into the room
She says, you are looking very well
Then she pokes and she pulls...
And says, if it hurts you, please tell.

Well, your heart is still beating...
And your pulse is very strong
Your blood pressure is elevated...
Your cholesterol is all wrong!

There is protein in your kidney.
And your feet, they still swell
We could change your medications...
Just to see if you'd do well!

Something different the next time,
And it surely will be good.
We'll contact some other Doctors...
They'd make you well if they could!

Come back next week to Cardiology
There we must be very brief
Well, the Doctor didn't know it,
But it was a sweet relief.

You must go home now and rest often,
Be sure you get plenty of exercise.
Then we'll see you back in two weeks,
There, we'll give you more advice.

That poem was a turning point for me. Martha had given me a gift more valuable than the poem and her confidence. She helped me see that a patient is more than their medical history and the status of their disease. Behind all of that was a person with hopes and dreams for their future; a person with fears about how or even if they can attain those dreams.

Our doctor-patient relationship changed. At each subsequent visit I made sure to ask about her writing and she looked forward to sharing her poems. In all she gave me five of her poems - each one telling me a little more about herself as a person, and partly how it felt to be a patient.

It was near the end of my residency training when she gave me the hand-made hot pad. It is of a purple quilted fabric with three flower designs on one side. It's a bit misshapen - not a perfect square and the stitching was done unevenly, by hand. I have kept it all these years to remind myself of Martha and to remember the real gift she gave me - the insight to being a better doctor.

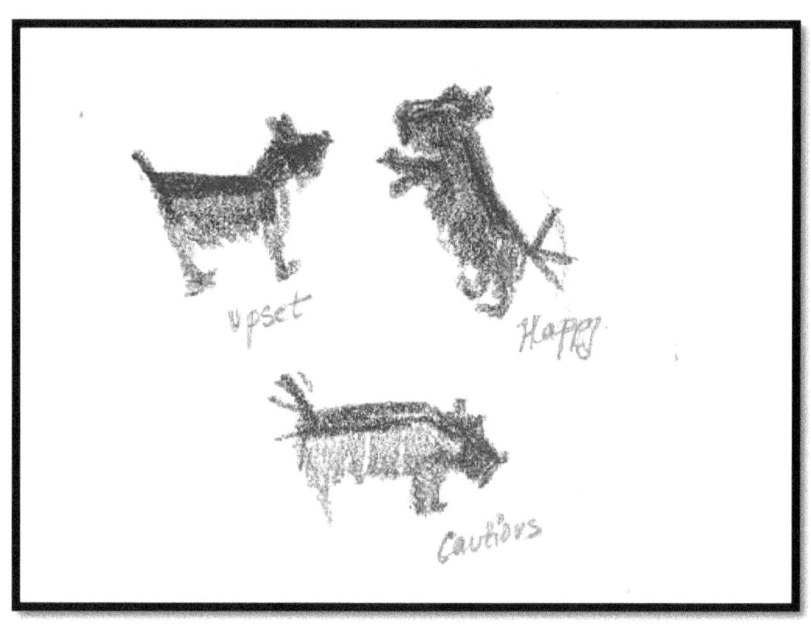

Feelings are Fleeting - watercolor & charcoal by Prasanna Menon, MD

It's Cooper Time

By Michael E. Day, MD

Some may call it meditation time. Some people may practice yoga. For some it may be doing biofeedback. For others it may entail listening to relaxing music. For me, I could call it dog time.

What I'm talking about is the time that many of us, and should be most of us, spend during the day collecting our thoughts, quit focusing on what we have to do at that moment, and just let our minds wander. For me it's often the time for reflection.

It usually starts in the morning when I get up out of bed and put on my clothes. I look up and see a pair of loving and longing eyes staring at me. Those eyes would belong to Cooper, my Brittany Spaniel. I know what he wants. It's time for his run with Dad. He's usually very patient, although so excited that the tail wags the rest of his body while I'm putting on my shoes. When I'm ready and I reach for the leash, he can no longer restrain himself and starts to run around and do flips in the air. This is his magical moment, the highlight of his day. We are ready to go take our run (for Cooper) and our mixed run/walk (for me.)

I really don't know who gets the most benefit from this time, me, or Cooper. But I know that without his insistence, I could very easily just put on the coffee, grab a newspaper or my iPhone and sit down in an easy chair instead of getting some exercise. Laziness comes easy to me, particularly at this stage of my life.

I have to admit, it's easier in Las Cruces, where I spend the winter months, to adhere to this morning routine. The sun shines virtually all the time. Rarely can I think of a good enough weather excuse on a southern New Mexico morning, although I may have to bundle up a bit. In Indiana, rain, snow, cold or just sloppy conditions make excuses easier during much of the year.

I have to admit, also, that I lucked into a great running and walking environment when I bought a place in Las Cruces. Right across the street from my house is a big desert sand hill, ideal for that morning exercise with Cooper. I think that hill was destined for further housing development, but there was a slowdown in construction a few years ago, much to my benefit. It has remained unoccupied and unbuilt for the three years that I have had my house here.

Once we get across the street, and through the corridor of tumble-weed stickers, I can release Cooper from his leash, and we can go at our own speeds. His is much faster than mine.

Through a combination of walking and jogging I can physically work off some of my anxiety, frustrations, and aggression. The physical activity is invigorating. The beauty of the morning seems to elevate me above the worry about society's problems. Somehow these concerns seem smaller, less acute. I see cars scurrying on the interstate and on Route 70, very small and far away from my viewpoint. I know that multitudes of people below in the valley are going about their daily lives and cares, but I am just observing, somehow outside of it all. This point of view puts my problems and concerns in a better perspective. I can concentrate on the far-off massive splendor of the Robledos, the sunrise over the Organs. I can dream and reflect. I can appreciate the beauty of the moment.

Cooper can concentrate on the smell of the jack rabbit that he will never catch. But hope springs eternal. And the joy is in the chase, in the journey.

Ideas suddenly pop into my brain. Thoughts seem to enter my ear, and I hope I can hold onto those ideas before they escape out of my other ear. Sometimes I have to hurry back to the house to get them down on paper before they vanish; or, more commonly these days, onto the "notes" section of my smart phone.

Various emotions materialize to me on our excursions. It seems like one of the first is always thankfulness that I can physically make my way up that hill. I know that not everyone my age, or some of any age, can make the trek up the hill, and see and appreciate the sights, and hear the sounds of the morning. It's something like my feelings these days on a golf course. I may not be able to hit the ball worth a darn, but then if I just step back and reflect for a moment and see the beauty of the course and its surroundings, and the fact that I can at least get out and play, I am thankful. Of course, given the quality of my golf game, I had better feel that way or else I would fall into despair!

On our walk/runs, just like with most exercise, my endorphins are stimulated. Happy hormones abound. The cares and cautions about worldly affairs seem to diminish some. My wife has learned that this is the best time to ask me for a favor, such as "can I buy some new clothes?" I am less likely to raise my eyebrows and ask questions about our financial status. I'm more likely to say something like "OK, honey, whatever you'd like."

Another feeling that seems to pop up is a sense of awe. Looking at the huge surrounding sky, as well as the surrounding mountains, I feel my own sense of smallness in this place. I feel happy to just be here and be able to appreciate it.

The final feeling is a sort of weird sense of responsibility. I need to share my blessings. This doesn't come from any sense of guilt, or any "requirements" imposed on me. It just feels good. I feel a need to help others appreciate their lives.

After coming back down the hill and back to my house, I am ready for that cup of coffee, and even a little inspired to write about my experience.

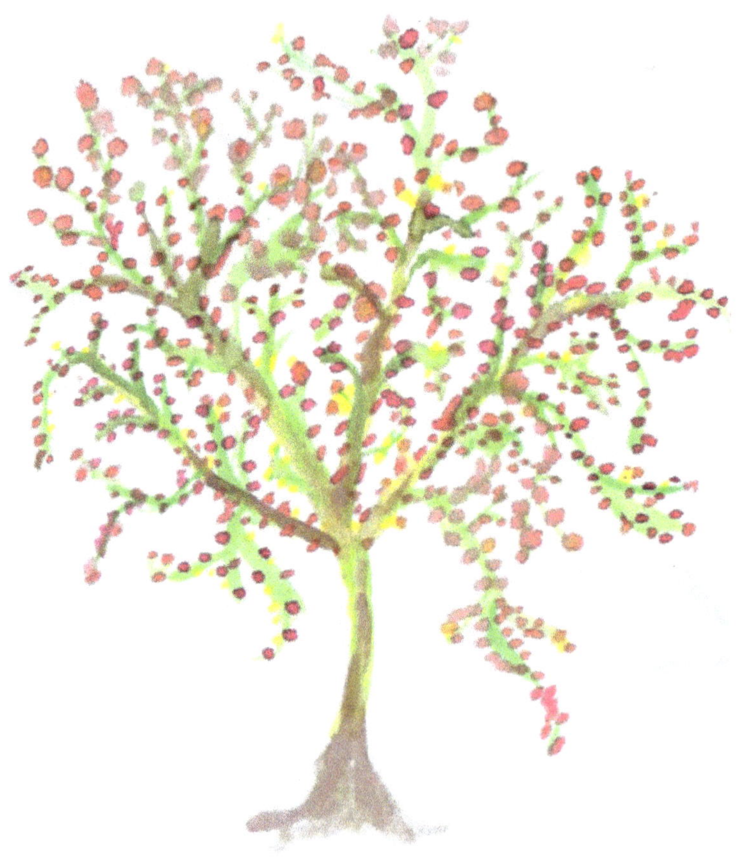

Imminent Spring Anew - watercolor by Charles E. Schwartz, MD

Imminent Spring Anew

By Charles E. Schwartz, MD

Today, third day of Spring,
(so they say),
so grey, overcast,
becomes raw, as dusk descends.

Nearly home,
I wind my way along Roosevelt Island's historical walk's
cherry tree-lined riverside promenade.

Drifting along, carried by this estuary's tide,
first, fresh flows south and down to the sea,
then, in complete about face,
north, propelled by the wave of saltwater heading inward,
downward then back, and homeward.

I briefly glance at the smattering of forlorn, wintered trees,
lifeless ghosts, still bearing wizened leaves of the season past,
clinging on, browned, lifeless.

But I am drawn to the resolute line of trees,
hugging the river's shore,
radiating life.

As winter wanes giving way to spring,
robust branches are brought low,
laden with buds,

grown swollen to near bursting,
green-leafed sepals out,
protective coronas circled around,
awaiting their precious cherry blossoms, tinted pink-red.

I begin to hear the warble of a jay,
hiding away from me,
it flashes in, then out of sight.
Now joined by other spring birds,
flitting tree-to-tree,
starting alone,
singing its song,
then joined, in twos and threes.

Suddenly, turning a corner,
I come upon buds
become the earliest of these precious blossoms,
sheltered within the University's quad.

A wondrous canvas unfolds before me,
blossoms in full bloom,
tinted pink and pastel hued,
living watercolors,
vibrantly seen, almost heard.
blossoms within reach of my fingers.

With joy they herald the arrival of Spring,
here,
then across the river,
and across the world.

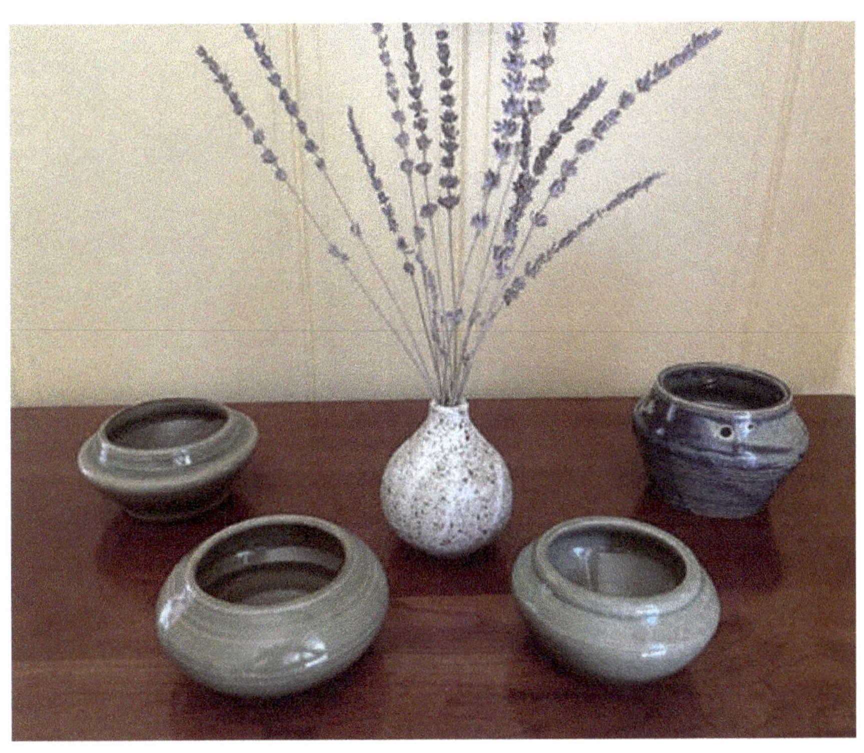

Four Bowls and White Vase - ceramics by Germaine L. Defendi, MD

Joy

By Cynthia A. Point, MD

From time to time,

I have seen you,

Silhouetted against

The darkening evening sky

Perched on top of the

Goal post, still and black.

I long to see you fly

And have missed it

Over and over again.

But last night, I saw

You spread your magnificent

Wings and saw your

Noble face as you glided

Across my path.

My heart soared.

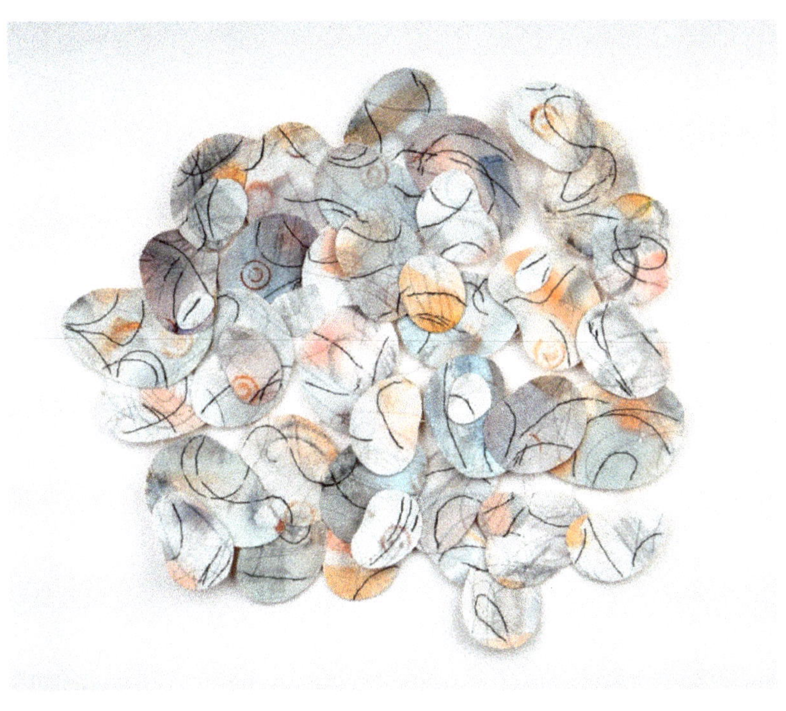

Convergence – mixed media by Jeanne Reisman, MD

CHAPTER TWO

Early Journeys

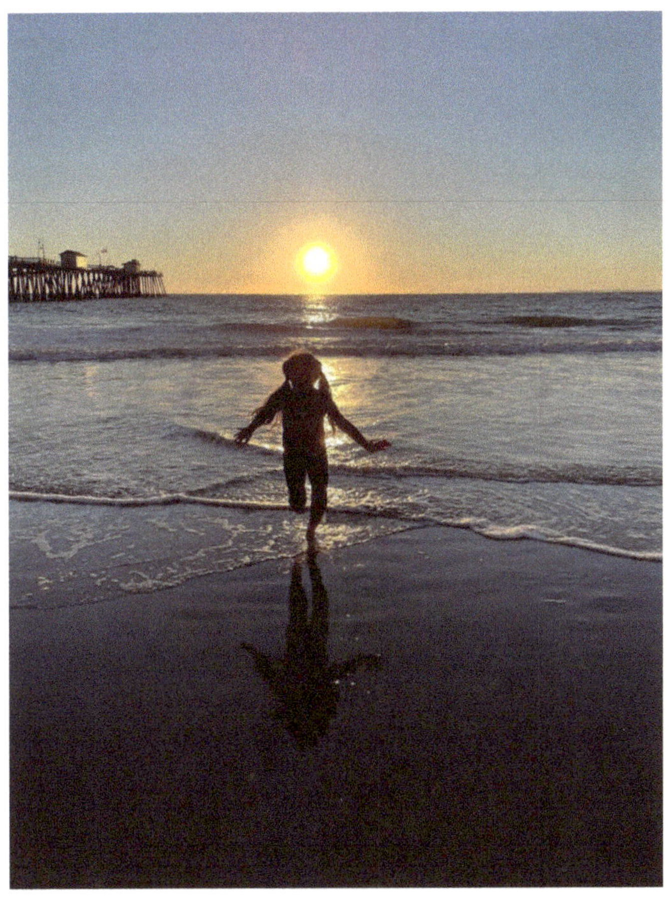

Emergence - photograph by Barbara Loeb, MD

Dad... Catch that ball!

By Scott Abramson, MD

One summer Sunday afternoon in 1957, when I was ten years old, my dad and I participated in a father-son softball game at the local Jewish community center. Now, this may not seem like a big deal, but in my family's history, this was unique. My dad had never participated in anything like this before or since. We had never even played catch together. First of all, Dad was much older than the other dads. He was forty-five when I was born. Secondly, Dad worked long hours, six days a week. He just didn't have the time to engage in throwing a baseball or camping trips or bike rides with his son. Thirdly, well...Dad was a klutz. And finally, I honestly don't think Dad knew how to relate to all this stuff. Growing up in a broken home, he was "raised" by various relatives. He had no father figure as a role model.

That's why it was so incredible to see my father on that Sunday afternoon, standing rather uncomfortable in Piedmont Park's right field. Sure enough, in the second inning, an easy pop fly gets hit into right field, straight at Dad. My father stood there with his glove outstretched. He seemed bewildered. He had no idea what to do. His arms made a few futile, helpless motions, then the ball hit his head and dropped pathetically to the ground. The other dads and their sons chortled with laughter. Dad was not hurt. The whole thing didn't seem to bother him at all. But I was devastated. In front of all my friends, my dad had just made a "spaz" of himself. (That is the unfortunate word we used back then.)

I was embarrassed,

I was humiliated.

And painfully, of my own father, I was ashamed.

And yet, just then, strangely enough, another emotion then flooded over me. I'm not sure why. Maybe it was because, deep down, Dad knew he would probably make a spectacle of himself. In his entire life, he had probably never even tossed a baseball. Yet on this day, for me... he stepped up to the plate. And at that very moment the softball careened off his befuddled body, I felt a wave of love rush into my heart. At that moment, I do not think I have ever loved that man more than I did that Sunday afternoon in Piedmont Park.

Over sixty years have passed since that summer afternoon. I can still see Dad now, standing helplessly in right field, awaiting a softball he would never catch. And as it is with so many recollections of childhood, with each passing year, those bittersweet memories become softer, sweeter, and more gracious in the heart.

On the Air with Code Blue

By David C. Hurwitz, MD

As a child, before the Dodgers came to Los Angeles in 1958, I used to enjoy the rare opportunity to just lie back and listen to *The Major League Game of the Day*, when all the legendary heroes of my youth were actively playing the game. You can imagine my consternation to find that my regular broadcast at San Francisco General was not baseball, but a code blue. It often went as follows:

"Would anyone have an EKG machine not in use bring it to Ward thirty-five." (Uh Oh, we have a problem on Ward thirty-five.)

Ten minutes would pass and then the announcement would come:

"Anyone having a Bird Respirator not in use please bring it to Ward thirty-five." (Things are getting worse.)

Inevitably after these two announcements:

"Code Blue Ward thirty-five, Code Blue Ward thirty-five" (The Code Blue Team would be dispatched.)

Sometime after the Code Blue had been called, we would hear:

"Father Scott, Father Scott, please come to Ward thirty-five." (The hospital chaplain has been called; this is not good.)

Then finally and all too often:

"Would the Ward X attendant come to Ward thirty-five?" (You can probably guess that the Ward X attendant was the mortuary attendant.)

Here I was, a medical student going on about my business, examining a patient and working the encounter into a spectacularly long history and physical document, and I had been witnessing, albeit second-hand, to the passing of a life. A profound circumstance, even though I was not actually there.

45

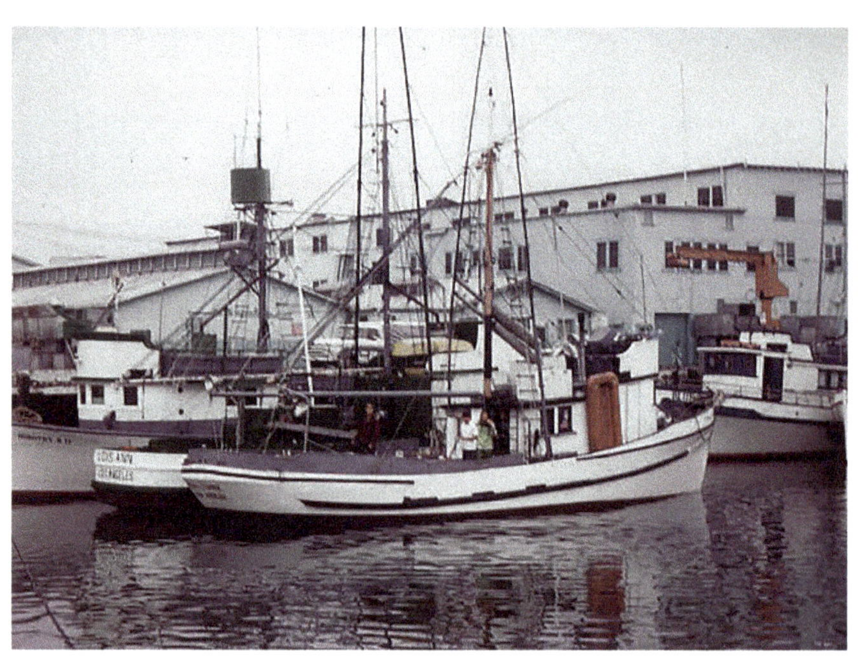

The Tuna Clipper 1969 - photograph by Peter M. McGough, MD

The Tuna Clipper

By Peter M. McGough, MD

SINBAD'S

It all started at Sinbad's Restaurant on the Santa Monica Pier in the Spring of 1969, when I was in my junior year at Redondo Union High School in Southern California. I neither liked washing dishes nor aspired to a higher position in any restaurant, but I was up to my elbows washing pots and pans and prepping for the cooks on a sunny Saturday afternoon. My dad, known to his friends as Babe, was out front in the bar serving drinks to the early afternoon regulars. During the week I went to school and did my homework at the library just next to the Redondo Beach pier, and each weekend I got to drive with my dad up to Sinbad's where I pulled in one dollar and thirty-five cents an hour, the minimum wage at the time. I liked the people but hated the job.

That afternoon, a long-time friend of my dad's, Red Dougherty, came into the bar and sat down looking dejected. When my dad asked him what was up, Red (who owned and operated a sixty-five-foot northern trawler named The Tuna Clipper) shared that his deck hand had just gotten tossed into jail and apparently would be there for some time. Red was just getting his boat ready for the upcoming tuna season, and it was sitting up on stands for repairs and painting down in the San Pedro Harbor. Each day without help would cost him money and time. He asked Babe if he knew anyone who might be interested.

"You can ask my kid. He's in the back washing dishes". Red asked if I had any experience on boats. "Nope, but he's a hard worker and likes the ocean".

One beer later Red was standing next to me back in the kitchen where I was leaning over a sink full of dishes.

"You interested in fishing for tuna this summer" he asked.

"Do I have to wash any dishes?" I shot back.

"Just your own" Red said and grinned. I said I'd take the job.

There were several ways to fish for tuna back then. One was on a purse seiner, which involved catching tuna in nets. Another used lines of fishermen side by side who caught the tuna individually with a pole and line. The Tuna Clipper was designed to catch tuna by trolling several lines that ran behind near the surface and used hydraulic reels to haul the fish in.

There are also many kinds of tuna including skipjack, yellowfin, bigeye and bluefin. The most prized tuna was albacore, which was the basis for the commercial tuna industry. Albacore swim in large schools that are highly migratory. Back when my dad fished tuna, they could be found down off the coast of Baja California where it was warm and sunny. As I would soon find out, the tuna had since moved their feeding grounds considerably north.

SAN PEDRO

San Pedro back in the 1960s had a thriving commercial fishing fleet. I spent a few Spring weekends helping Red on the boat. Then, when school let out, I worked with him pretty much every day. The first job was to scrape the entire boat, especially the hull, caulking and repainting it. Red spent a lot of his time making sure the equipment, starting with the diesel engine, was in working order. This took most of the time getting ready for sea, and once the Tuna Clipper was eased back into the water, we could finish the work on the deck equipment and the cabin.

The cabin was small. Walking through the aft hatch of the cabin there was a compact galley with a table, stove, and sink. Passing just forward there was a bunk for two that opened into the forward steering compartment. Across from the bunks, accessed from the steering compartment, was a closet sized room that had once been the "head" or bathroom but had been retrofitted into an electronics room (I was to find out where we were supposed to relieve ourselves later.)

Back on deck you accessed the upper control station via a ladder. During good weather, when we weren't working, this was a great place to be. In the center of the deck, just behind the mast, was the hatch down into the storage hold where we would keep tons of ice and, when they were caught, the tuna.

Outfitting and stocking the Tuna Clipper for sea took about a week. This included getting my gear for fishing and especially for rough weather. I brought my guitar and some books aboard, which brought an "Oh Jesus" and an eye roll from Red.

Finally, we were ready to launch. After saying good-bye to family and friends Red picked me up in his car and we climbed aboard the boat and let loose the mooring lines and headed out of San Pedro Harbor. Once outside the entrance to the harbor, Red gave a big sigh and tossed my books over the side. "I need your complete attention on the boat at all times." Luckily, he stored my guitar in a locker.

I had worked since age twelve, but never this hard. It prepared me for the later demands of medical training. It also created a strong sense of self-reliance, independence, and a better understanding of the risks in life.

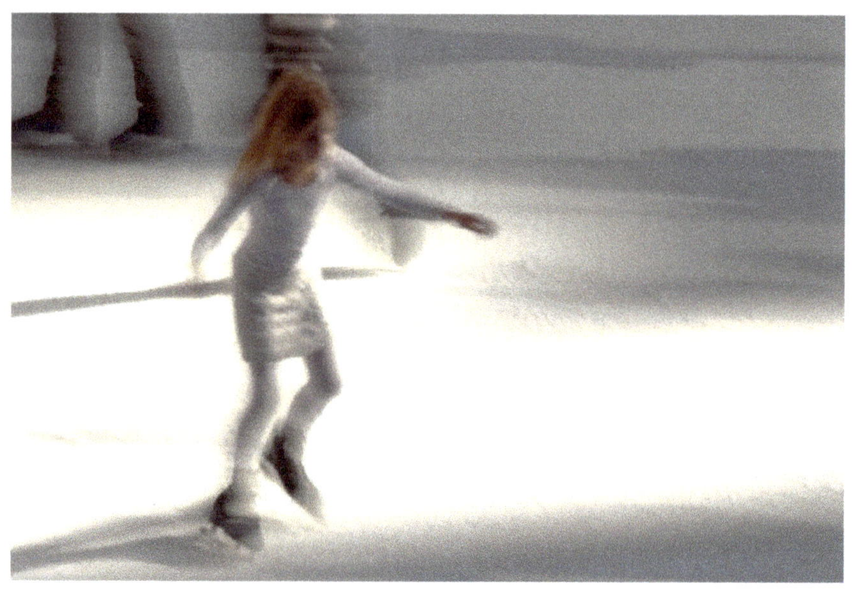

Ice Skating at the Rockefeller - photograph by Grace D. Bandow, MD

Tipping Point

By Barbara Loeb, MD

At 3 I learned to hop on one foot - my mother cheering

At 8 she freed my hand - I glided gracefully across the ice

At 13 - yes 13 - she let go of my bike handlebars – off I went

At 28 I jogged cautiously with my baby strapped to my belly

At 42 I hiked a narrow rocky path on the edge of a cliff

At 52 I ziplined weightless through the clouds across an abyss

At 67 I learned to hop on one foot - my grandchildren cheering

At every stage, we find our balance

to cautiously venture to the tipping point

and draw back at exactly the right moment.

If we misstep, we find ways to recover

with more resilience than when we began.

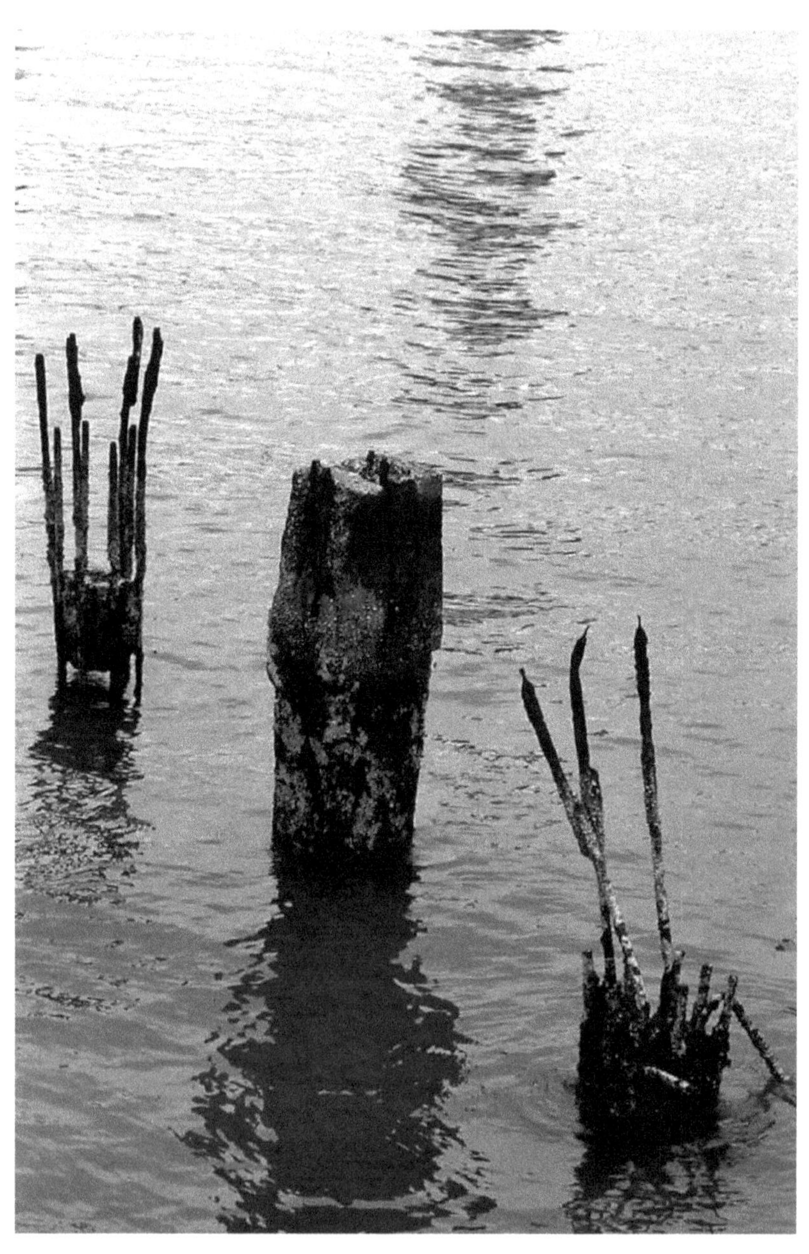

Reflections with Pier - photograph by Cynthia A. Point, MD

My Bicycle Trips to School

By LoAn Nguyen, MD

Dalat, Viet Nam, is a relatively small city located in Vietnam's southern central highlands; it had the population of about sixty thousand in the mid-1960s during the time of this story. It is known for its temperate climate, which allows the area to be a big producer of fresh vegetables, flowers, and fruits such as strawberries, avocados, persimmons, etc. The town is also famous for golf courses, romantic lakes, waterfalls, green pine hills and verdant valleys. I grew up in the tiny village of Xanh Rang, that is located about nine miles from the center of the city.

After completing elementary school, I took the entrance exams and was admitted to the only all-girls public school for middle and high school, Bui Thi Xuan. That school was equivalent to highly competitive STEM magnet schools in the U.S. today. Unfortunately, Bui Thi Xuan school was located about twelve miles from our home. Adding to the challenge, I was the only kid from the village who would be attending. Many of my contemporaries stopped school to help their families with farming; others who failed the entrance exam had to attend private schools, which were about eight miles from the village.

Buses or other transportation did not exist in such a remote place, so my choices for getting to the school broke down to either walking or riding a bicycle. The former was nearly impossible in terms of time and energy for a young girl. Despite these issues, my parents and I knew we had to devise a practical way for me to attend that prestigious school.

I will never forget how my dad sacrificed his time and strength biking me to and from school every day. It was quite an arduous trip, on a bad road with many hills. Some of the hills were so steep that Dad had to get off the bike and push us ahead. He would not let me off the bike, insisting that my energy be saved for learning. Of course, I silently wished I were a bit lighter so that he would not have to push as hard! A child's heart is innocent and tender, so watching the beaded sweat drops on my dad's face made my heart ache. The only sensible thing I could do was to use the time to memorize my lessons and finish up any homework; by the time we arrived at the school, I would be totally ready.

My Dad's love was indescribable at the time, and still is for me today. His was a marvelous gift that motivated me and built the resilience I needed to eventually enter the unimaginable world that lay in store for me many years later. His kindness, vision, sacrifice, and dedication to my education made me who I am and into what I was to become.

How to Ride a Bike

By Barbara Loeb, MD

To learn how to ride a bike you need to own one. That was my first problem. I grew up in inner-city Chicago where it wasn't common for young children to have bicycles. Riding them on the street was unsafe. Besides, they were expensive, at least fifty dollars. Most folks living in our neighborhood couldn't afford to spend that kind of money on a non-essential purchase, especially when the average mid-1960s weekly wage was only one hundred twenty-five dollars. In our family, my mother relied on irregularly paid child support of thirty dollars per week, rarely paid alimony of ten dollars per week and the good graces of friends to support my sister Teri and me.

On weekends my mom would take us to the parks and beaches that lined Lake Michigan. I'd see people riding down the eighteen-mile bike path and pictured what it would be like to be able to be one of those carefree riders. Somehow, I knew with certainty one day I would be one of them. I just didn't know when or how.

It was in June 1967 when I was thirteen and graduating from eighth grade that my mother surprised me with my first bicycle. She had been saving up S&H green stamps that were given to customers with their grocery purchases at the National Tea Company store and gasoline at the Standard Oil station. I can still remember the taste of the glue as I licked the stamps and pasted them into books. I always volunteered for this task using my tongue in place of a sponge to wet them because I liked that taste.

You needed twenty-six books of stamps for one bicycle. Each book contained twenty-four pages of fifty points or five dollars' worth of stamps per page, in denominations of ten, twenty-five, and fifty points. You had to spend one hundred and twenty dollars to fill one book. Doing the math, mom had spent three thousand, one hundred and twenty dollars on groceries and gas to get enough stamps for that one bike. This took her almost three years.

On that day in June, I opened a brown cardboard box to find a turquoise and white Schwinn bicycle with chrome handlebars ready for assembly. It had one speed "forward." It was called a coaster because you coast forward and then back pedal to engage the brakes. After quickly putting it together, we headed out to the bike path. I was ecstatic and filled with anticipation about mounting my new steed.

I glanced down the long path and at the bikers passing by. How hard could this be? After a few brief instructions from mom, I began trying a variety of techniques. First, I put my right leg over the center bars of the frame and placed my right foot on the pedal. Then scooted forward trying to balance and get my left foot onto the left pedal. I tried this repeatedly but couldn't quite get my foot all the way up into the correct position. Then mom held the bike steady while I got onto the seat. She gave me a little push and then let go but that didn't work too well either. She had to catch me as I began to fall to one side. Finally, we gave up for the day. We repeated this attempt multiple times over the next week. I felt like I was gradually getting closer to success, but I had a little further to go.

It was on a perfect balmy Saturday. We arrived early to give us more time to practice. I was ready, full of energy and determination that this would be the day. After several scooting failures, I propped myself onto the seat with mom's help. She said "ok, let's do it." I took a deep breath;

she began to run by my side holding the handlebars. With the momentum built she loosened her grip and let go. I balanced perfectly and off I went.

I had an overwhelming sense of freedom, greater than any other I can remember. I was filled with supernatural power. At that moment, I felt I could do anything. At the same time, I experienced a surge of deep appreciation for this incredible gift my mother had given me. She always made sure I had things that other children took for granted. Not only the bike, but the ability to fly away.

Fifty-five years later I still ride my bike every day if the weather permits. Sometimes on the same path. But no matter where I ride, it's always with that same empowerment and gratitude.

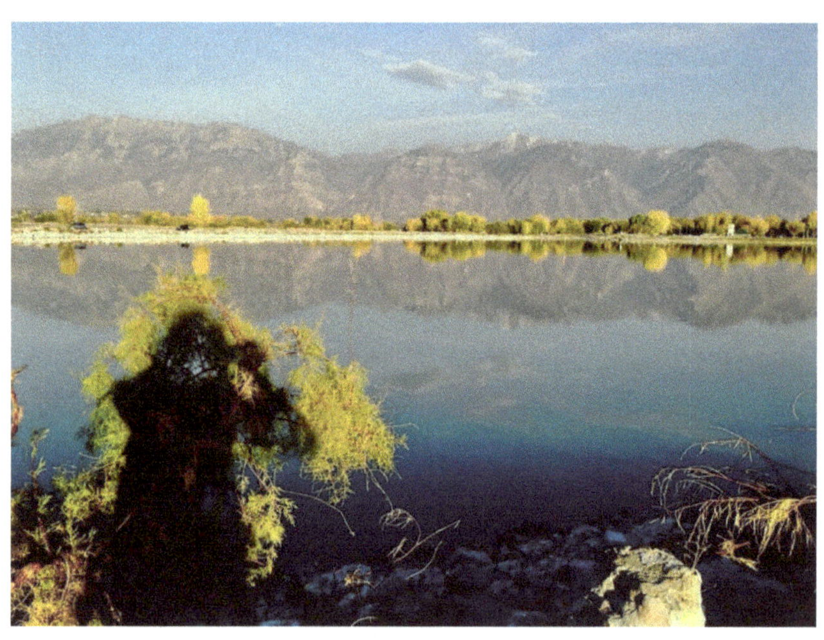

Snapshot - Lake Utah - photograph by Barbara Loeb, MD

Childhood Memories Sixty Years On

By Tom E. Norris, MD

Childhood memories do not flow,
From start to end, like video.
Instead, snapshots, a slice of life.
Some happy, some sad, some filled with strife.

As the years pile up from here to there.
I grow older, wiser, lose my hair.
Instead of focus, crystal clear.
Now edges fuzz, the scenes do blur.

From sequences, all lined up and straight.
To random pictures, through the gate.
From sharp edged photos every day,
To fuzz soft scenes, like by Monet.

Let's keep the happy and the good.
The smiles from our old neighborhood.
Let's lose the pain, the strife, the fear.
So, childhood memories improve each year.

CHAPTER THREE
What Patients Teach Us

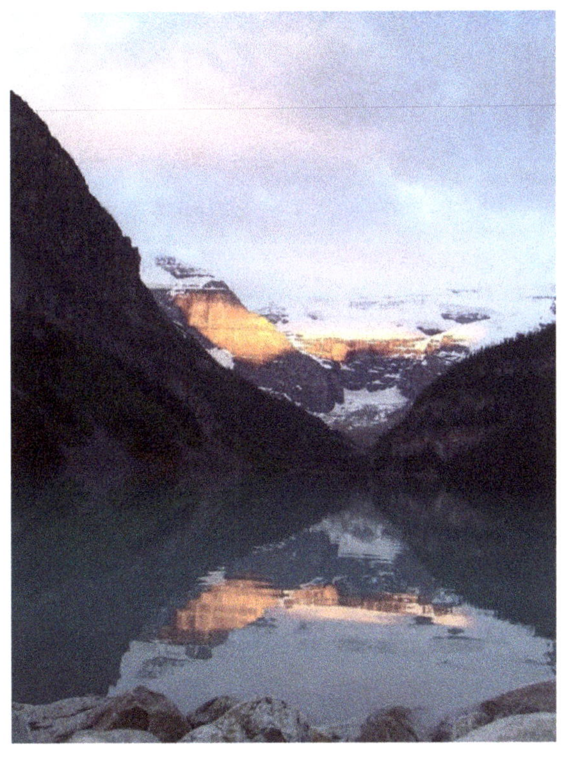

Dawn at Lake Louise - photograph by Cynthia A. Point, MD

Elegy for Josie

By Jill Silverman, MD

One summer day, the air palpably thick,
I first met Josie, a hard living gal.
A scarf wrapped around her sinewy neck,
Her hair a tangled nicotine yellow.

She was rubbing her face repeatedly.
I noticed a fading mark on her cheek.
Our eyes met somewhat uncomfortably.
Should I ask? No, not a good idea. So
I looked away
And we talked of other things.

Diabetes - right now not doing well.
Out of work - unable to buy her meds.
"Jimmy will help me. Probably he will."
Jimmy her guy. "Maybe my only friend."

The winter brought in Josie sporting shades.
I started to inquire casually.
Her head turned. She was trying to evade.
Should I ask? No, not a good idea.

So, I looked away again.
We talked of other things.

She was working. "Jimmy's working too."
They would fight, she said, but always made up.
She'd been with Jimmy since she was fourteen.
"No one done ev'r loved me n'erly so much."

Summer passed and she stopped coming around.
I thought she had probably moved along.
That was common among the trailer crowd-
A life of running from or searching for.

It was another blazing summer day.
Like many others we would suffer through.
A quick stop for a biscuit and gravy.
I grabbed a local weekly to peruse.

I must have gasped -as people stared.
"Woman Killed by Boyfriend in Trailer Park"
I looked away once again. My eyes teared.
Too late - no chance to talk of other things.

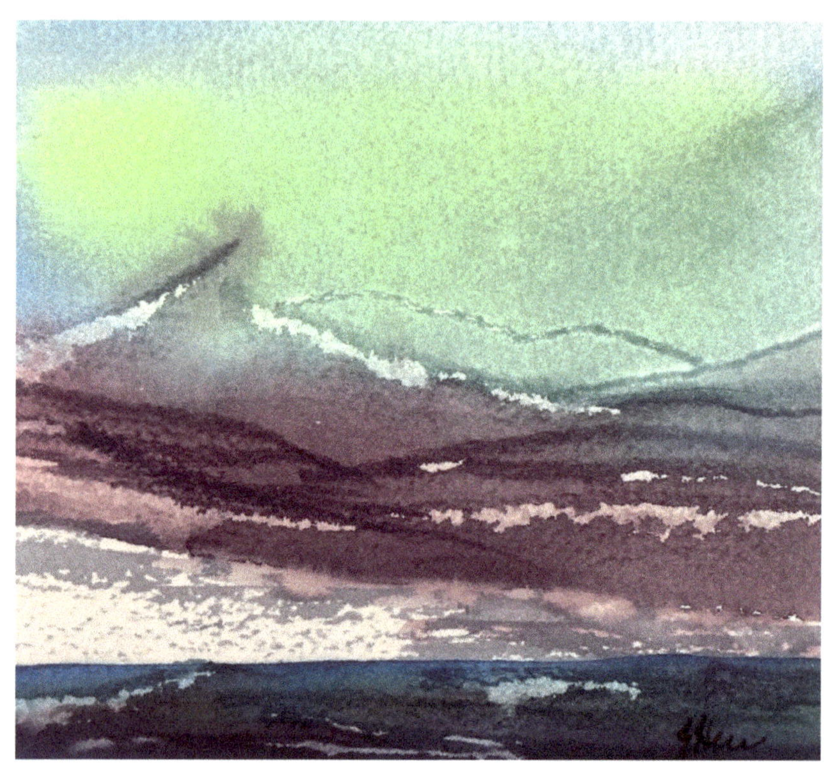

Ocean Mountain Sky - watercolor by Jan L. Herr, MD

My Teacher Patient

By LoAn Nguyen, MD

Glancing at my list of afternoon patients, it looked to be a busy day; but something quite atypical caught my eye. A new patient's name on the schedule jumped out. I recognized an unusual Vietnamese name, P.L. She appeared to be someone who had influenced my life in a far-distant time and place. I was intensely curious and excited to meet this new patient.

Her name conjured up treasured memories of my 9th-grade high school philosophy teacher, a very beautiful, intelligent young woman in her mid-twenties who was admired and beloved. We saw her as an ideal role model, someone we would want to emulate when we grew up.

I have absolutely no recollection of what she taught me in philosophy. But I remember with utmost clarity and joy the last ten minutes of each class, when she rewarded our diligence and obedience by reading a segment from Charlotte Bronte's *Jane Eyre*. By this, she opened the vast world of Western literature to me, which grew into my lifelong enjoyment of classic literature, especially with its insights into humanity.

P.L. was the first patient who arrived for my afternoon session. Although she was much altered, I recognized her immediately. I felt a pang in my chest upon seeing how my idol had changed so much since I last saw her. She was now a middle-aged woman in her fifties, humbly dressed. There was an aura of subdued quietness about her, but I still saw the kind, vibrant look in her eyes. She did not recognize me as her former student, which was not a surprise since I was a student among the fifty all-girl classrooms.

We quickly expressed our amazement and unexpected pleasure of reconnecting after so many years. Our discussion then focused on her past medical history and preventive care. Her only medical problem was chronic insomnia. As I began to learn more about P.L.'s life, I felt an enormous sense of privilege and good fortune in the opportunity to take care of my favorite teacher.

Five years after the fall of Saigon, she arrived in the U.S. as one of the "boat people" who escaped the communist regime seeking freedom in America. She and her family resettled in Washington, D.C. With limited English, she worked in a local library stacking books. In her free time, she wrote a column, *Laughing with Ms. L.*, for a local Vietnamese magazine. She seemed content with her new life.

Over the following ten years, her insomnia continued to be somewhat troublesome. We explored the possibility of post-traumatic stress disorder, but she denied any intrusive symptoms typical for it. Cognitive Behavioral Therapy, sleep specialist evaluation, and sleeping medications were tried without much success. She never expressed frustration or distress about her insomnia.

One day I received a phone call from her husband telling me that P.L. was hospitalized; she had made a suicide attempt using over-the-counter medications. Hearing the shocking news, I reflected on our recent encounters. I asked myself, "What did I miss? Should I have..." I was profoundly sad; had I let my favorite teacher and her family down? Later that day I visited her at the psychiatric ward. P.L. was in typical form: pleasant, unassuming. She showed no signs of being depressed or troubled by what had happened. She simply told me matter-of-factly that she did not feel the need to continue living. When I asked if she would try again, she said that the suicide failure meant that her fate was to live out her reincarnation. After discharge, she declined psychiatric follow-up. She continued with the medication for a few months then discontinued it on her own.

I continued to be her primary care physician for another five years or so. In each visit, I diligently probed for changes in her mental health. She faithfully adhered to all preventive recommendations. She appeared to be physically healthy and content with her life.

Then awful news arrived. The saddest day of my medical career came when I received a call from her husband, who had found her peacefully passed away while taking a nap. There were no notes or empty bottles; nothing obvious had changed before her last nap. Her husband felt she had willed herself to die.

Words cannot describe the sorrow of losing my beloved childhood teacher. Decades before, she taught me to love literature, opening vast spaces of human emotion and psychology over centuries of time. On many occasions I have expressed my gratitude for the impact she had on my education and my life. But she would never know how her death would teach me the profound humility of being a physician when treating patients with mental illness.

As primary care physicians, we have knowledge, tests, and specialists to help arrive at diagnoses to treat or ease physical suffering. But secret mental anguish and contradictions of the psyche do not yield readily to diagnosis and treatment. The depth of suffering for patients with mental illness is often beyond our comprehension or reach. I thought I was competent to treat my teacher because I spoke her language, understood her culture, and could draw upon superb medical training that had served me and my patients so well for years. Yet behind her pleasantries and ostensibly happy demeanor surely lurked a remote untouchable pathos which proved to be her final philosophy lesson. Her death reinforces for me that each patient has a very complex set of values, beliefs, and coping mechanisms forged by what life has brought to them. Looking into a patient's troubled mind is to gaze at light from a distant galaxy, for what we see is a long-past mirage of reality.

Wait for it...

By Susan Boiko, MD

Nine o'clock in the morning and I was already behind. Evaluations over my career as an HMO dermatologist had always been the same: the patients love you; the staff love you, but could you work a little faster?

The electronic medical record on this patient had a diagnosis column filled with variations on themes of mania, depression, psychosis. I took a deep breath and let it out slowly before entering the room. As I opened the door I saw a greying, middle aged woman sitting with hunched posture at on the edge of the exam table, clad in a plain beige knit sweater and beige slacks. She looked towards the door handle, not meeting my gaze even after I cheerfully called out her name and sat with the computer turned so she could read along with me as I typed.

"I'll be the driver and you be the passenger - have a look at the windshield (computer screen) and please correct me if I'm writing or saying anything wrong." In this manner I had gotten grammatical corrections from retired English professors, medical record shortcut tips from medical people, even a few grins as autocorrect "helped" with some bizarre suggestion. But this patient sat silently, her gaze above the giant screen.

Normally, my comment on her clothing- "that looks like a really cozy sweater you have on" would get a comment about the impulse purchase on that trip to Scotland, her mother's closet, or something – anything - I could riff on to build a bridge between us, a common interest, but my words fell flat as she stared over the computer screen at the exit door with that faraway look.

"How can I help you with your skin?" I pushed the computer aside to face her.

Silently, she removed her sweater. Shallow sores on both arms told the story of skin picking. Already mentally planning a subsequent visit where I could see all her skin, I was giving my canned speech about what we then called neurotic excoriations as I examined her hands, telltale dried blood under her fingernails.

I paused here and there to see if she would add any comments. None. I talked about comforting habits that are harmful to skin as she was showing me her arms. "I'd like to suggest some simple strategies"- our HMO chiefs had drilled us to use the word *strategy* as that was a metric by which patients would judge us on an after-visit questionnaire, "did the doctor share any strategies."

I gently placed her hands back in her lap and finished with, "so think about cutting your nails as short as mine, smoothing them with a nail file so no jagged edges, and when you want to pick, massage Vaseline into the areas with your fingertips instead."

I took a step towards the door, as I said my exit line, "Is there anything else important that we haven't talked about today?" I was mentally girding myself for the complaint from the next patient about my lateness, when I finally heard her low, clear voice and saw her looking straight at me.

"I was raped ten years ago, and I never told anyone."

Any lingering worry about future patient wrath vanished as I inwardly marveled at what strength it took her to trust me - ME - over ten years of predecessors. I opened the door and sang out to my assistant,

"Melinda, please come in here and sit with Ms. A. I need to call her primary care doctor right now."

I never have gotten any faster. And even now when a patient, a family needs that time, I will say to the next patients, "Thanks for waiting. It might sound hard to believe, but there can be emergencies in Dermatology, too!"

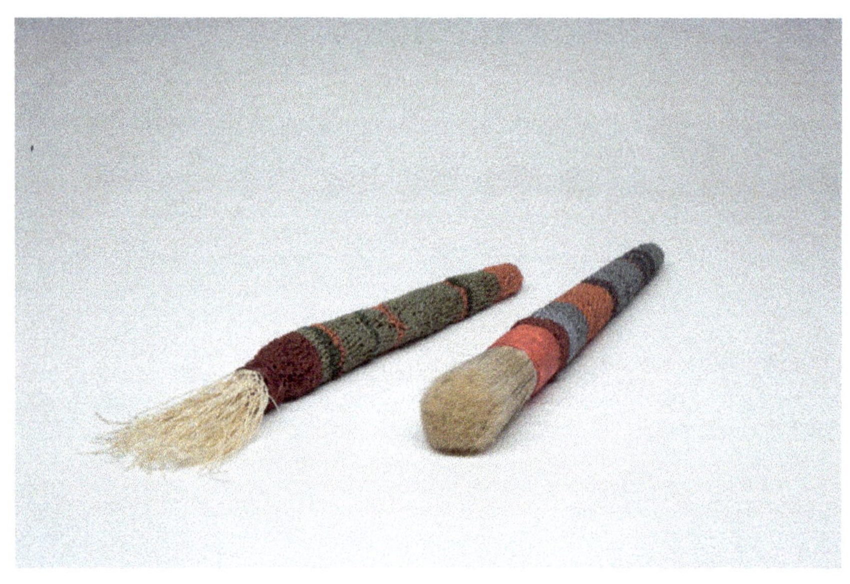

Rena's Brush - fiber sculpture by Jeanne Reisman, MD

Doctors' Stories

By John Orzano, MD

"Doctor, it's Mr. P. on the phone. It's about his wife."

"I'll be right there," I said.

"Do you need Mrs. P.'s chart?" I shook my head from side to side.

I had known Mr. and Mrs. P. and their two grammar school girls for at least five years. The family must have been one of my first twenty-five families in my practice. I remember the first evening Mr. and Mrs. P. came in. He introduced his wife. "This is my wife," he said. "She has MS." I thought she looked fine. She was short like him, with a smile on her face, talking and walking fine.

I picked up the phone: "Yes, Bob."

"It's Kate. I think she's gone," Mr. P. answered. "The kids are at school." There was silence on the phone. I tried to think of what to say. It's for the best is what I felt, but somehow, I couldn't say that, so I said I'd be right over.

My nurse and receptionist looked at me. The office was full of patients but getting over there was all I could think of doing. He knew I would come. I had even given him my home telephone number in case I wasn't in the office. I didn't do that for every patient. I admired Mr. P. for the way he took care of his wife. She always came first. He would do whatever he could to make her comfortable. He took care of the girls. He would go to their school events. Sometimes I couldn't figure out how he could manage it all. It was not only the physical strain but also the emotional aspects of the situation. When he brought his sick kids to the office, he was always optimistic and upbeat, with a smile on his face, despite what it must have been like at home.

"Thanks for coming doctor," Mr. P. said as I got to the house.

I think I put my arm on his shoulder, but I'm not sure. I mumbled something. Again, I don't remember.

"Come this way," he said, and he led me into the living room, where his wife was lying on the couch, barely filling a small blanket. Her weight was below ninety pounds without a doubt. The skin on her face was pulled taut over her cheekbones. Her eyes were closed.

Unable to say anything, I went closer and performed a ritual which still makes little sense. You see, no one in medical school taught me how to do this, what to say or what to do. I reached into my black bag, took out my stethoscope, applying its metal head to her cold chest. I heard nothing, not a sound. As if I wasn't sure, I pressed my two middle fingers against her neck. I could only feel my own pulse. I stepped back, bowed my head, and made a sign of the cross.

There was a visiting nurse in the room. She choked. "Maybe I could have done something," she said. I could tell she was uncomfortable, but I felt relieved for Mrs. P. I couldn't tell how Mr. P felt. He started talking to me about how much helpful I had been. I said to him, "I hope I can take care of my wife, God forbid, just half as much as you took care of yours."

In Memory of John H.

By Betsy Strong, MD

John H. was one of my first clinic patients. He was thirty-five years old when I met him. He presented at the end of my clinic day with a headache which he thought was (and I initially believed to be) a sinus headache. Thinking he needed to follow me to get a prescription, he came from the exam room to my office. It was a small office with a large desk. He ran into the corner of the desk. I suddenly realized that he had a visual field cut - this was not a simple sinus headache! I sent him for an immediate CT scan. The scan showed a subarachnoid hemorrhage, bleeding in the brain. He was transferred to the hospital for emergency surgery which was performed quickly and successfully.

Several years later, I cared for him when he had a heart attack. In those days, before the era of hospitalists, we used to round in the hospital before clinic. I recall sitting at the bedside, counseling him regarding his habits. Despite what had happened, he continued to smoke two packs of cigarettes and drink one to two six-packs a day. His excuse: "as a contractor it's hard not to smoke or drink around the guys."

John was later diagnosed with obstructive sleep apnea. Wearing a positive pressure face mask at night normalized his elevated red blood cell count and grayish complexion. This treatment probably added years to his life. He was compliant with his aspirin and medications for blood pressure and cholesterol. He eventually retired and moved out of the area, only to return for his annual physicals. He would joke with me as to why he should bother giving up his habits. We wondered who would survive longer, as we were born in the same year. I later heard he was found dead in his home, cause undetermined. He was fifty-nine years old.

I am now on the eve of retirement after many years of clinical practice. I reflect on this remarkable relationship with a man who came from a very different walk of life, who was not always compliant with my recommendations; yet we managed to forge a trusting relationship that lasted for more than two decades. This amazing aspect, that of lasting, trusting interpersonal relationships, is what I loved most about medical practice, and it kept me going. And yes, even in this day and age, I would still encourage a serious premed to go into medicine.

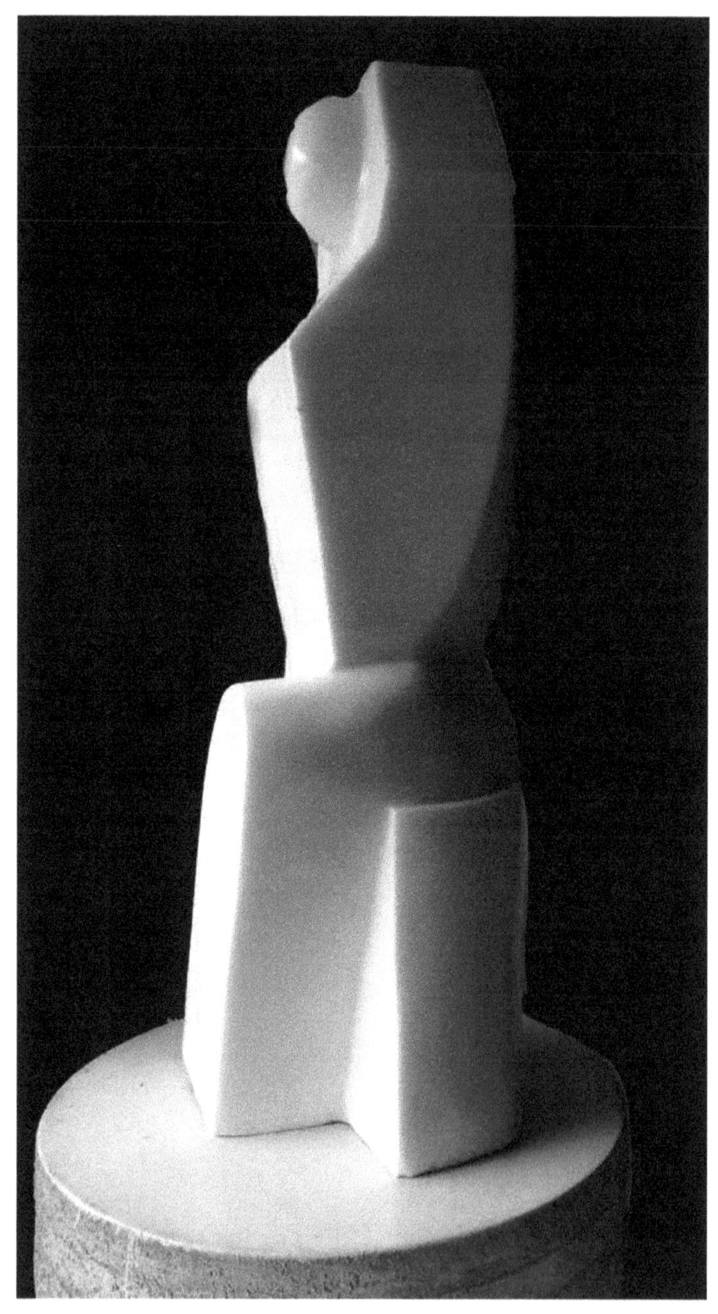

Sphinx #2 - marble by Kenneth Elconin, MD

And So Here Was S.

By Vahe A. Keukjian, MD

And so here was S.: a not-yet-fifty-year-old man of naturopathic persuasions; a family man, healthy all of his life until now. He rarely came to see me but finally did for a vague twinge in his abdomen. His examinations, labs and CT scan offered no clues. His colonoscopy showed a large cancer of the sigmoid colon. There was no trace of it in his family, nor any other reason to screen him for it before he was fifty.

When the surgeon went in to remove the tumor the next day, he found cancer spread thickly throughout the abdomen. He bypassed what he could, and S. made a remarkably fast recovery. S.'s wife told me she doubted he would agree to any further "conventional therapy". To our surprise, he tried a course of 5-FU and Leucovorin - all the chemotherapy we could offer, back then - till the treatment made him feel worse than the cancer did, and he swore off it. There were things he needed to do while he was still well enough, and he would not trade present living for the hope of longevity.

His end was really the beginning of our relationship. Success, therefore, would need some other measure than curing the patient, or the doctor doing something: rather, the doctor being someone. We arranged to get together monthly, to catch up. I would not press him about more chemo, or experimental drug trials. I had no idea how much this meant to him until he brought in cheesecake one day and thanked me for not abandoning him when he decided not to be treated. Noncompliance is, after all, the most mortal sin patients can commit against their doctors. For this, we throw them headlong from our practices, or else minutely chronicle their misdeeds to exculpate ourselves.

S. couldn't quite say no to shark cartilage or special diets, or to a chiropractor who claimed to fix colons by cracking necks; but he wasted no more time on those forlorn hopes than he had on chemotherapy. He was practical.

His attendance grew spotty: storms kept blowing, late into his life and pre-occupied him. He told me about these things matter-of-factly, without a trace of self-pity or pessimism or optimism, or any other kind of fantasy. It gave me the willies. I was on holy ground.

When he came back into the hospital with a bowel obstruction, the cancer was growing out through his previous abdominal incision. The surgeon had all he could do to find his way back into the peritoneal cavity and quickly finished the operation with little rearrangement inside. S. decided to enter hospice care at home. He returned to the hospital a couple of weeks later, vomiting, to die.

A nasogastric tube was inserted to keep his obstructed bowel decompressed and sucked out everything he tried to eat or drink. Pain medications made him feel too weird, he insisted not to use them until the very end. He had already said his goodbyes after the first surgery and, finding it too painful to repeat them, kept his family away; except for his mother, who sat with him, ready to run any errand, fulfill any request.

I visited S. on the hospice unit as often as I could. He asked me how much longer I thought he had, and I told him. "You've always been honest," he said. We tried to guess what colors would come out his nasogastric tube if he mixed watermelon and lime sherbet, or mochaccino and orange soda. Most of the time he was right on the money. Every moment was his, painful or otherwise.

The weekend he finally started to die in earnest, I happened to be on call. I stopped by at the end of my hospital rounds. His mother sat outside the room, reading, and watching. He had begun fading in and out - at the moment, he was in. "Mind if I hang around?" I asked. "Please," he said. I sat by his bed. We talked or not, as we liked. He reached out his hand and I took it. In that stillness, I had the curious sense not of ending, but of travelling; and soon, of arrival.

Some doctors would have prayed with S. I could not, though I am a believing Christian, as was he. Why not? I could give clever answers about holy silence and the theological tangles of intercessory prayer; but I don't really know why. Except to say that whatever we might have prayed about was already happening.

Finally, it was time to say goodbye, without sounding too much like I was crying - which I was. On the way out, I stopped to talk with his mother. "He's a good man," I said. "Yes, he is," she said. "He always was. He was a good boy and a good teenager and a wonderful man, always helping people, good to his family. He is suffering so much. He needs to go on." S. died the next day.

When people sometimes ask me about becoming a doctor, I advise them strongly against it, unless they believe in ghosts, and are willing to bear the burden of continual loss that practice entails. The dead never really leave us: they weigh softly and cumulatively on the present. Some doctors escape this by entering specialties rife with the healthy, but not most of us; not family doctors. We are intimate strangers in other peoples' lives, present in times of absolute risk and responsibility. For that privilege, we must take our lumps. Not just lawsuits or bad press, but standing at the foot of the cross, looking up at suffering and grace. When I am called a "gatekeeper" or a "healthcare provider," I think of

S., and of other ghosts: the way they are singing to me, shining, in the dark.

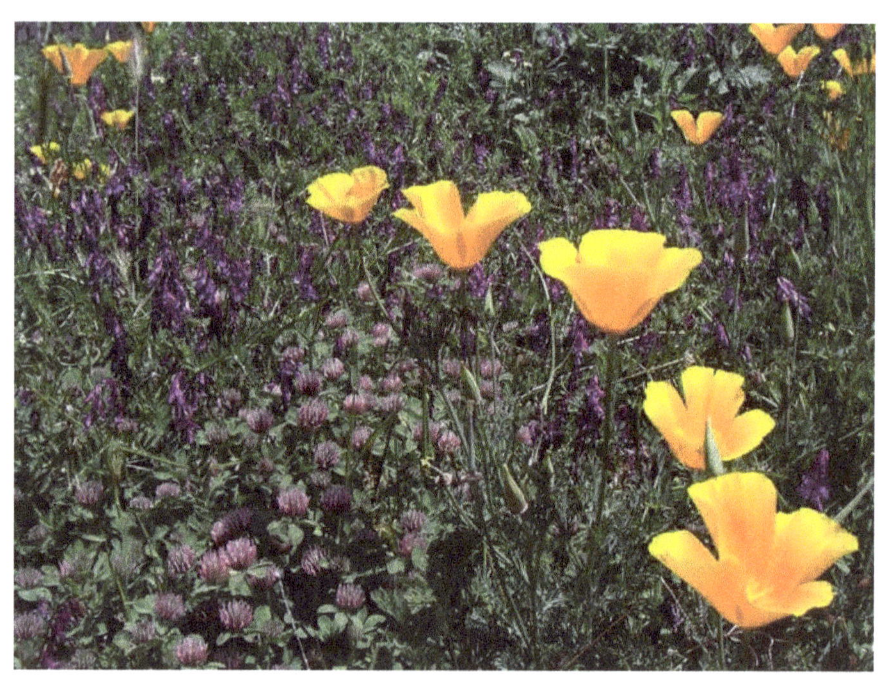

Wildflowers - photograph by Cynthia A. Point, MD

Begin Anew

By Cynthia A. Point, MD

When I picked up the phone that morning, she said "Jim (not his real name) died this morning. I washed his body, and dressed him in the clothes he had chosen, then called the Hospice Nurse, and now you." Laura (not her real name) sounded very fatigued and emotionally drained as she spoke. It had been a long hard process after his cancer diagnosis, and although we knew it was coming, it had been very difficult. I asked her how she was doing, and she told me how emotionally drained she was, and I thought of the enormous physical effort this had taken for her to do what she had told me. I asked her if she had injured herself, washing and dressing her husband's body, and she paused for a while, then said, "yes, but I can manage, I always do, and I needed to do this for him, I promised."

Laura had osteogenesis imperfecta, was about four feet tall with very long graceful hands, long brown hair, and needed a special surround custom walker to navigate her world. She had a special wry sense of humor and spoke with a slight accent. She had broken her bones so many times in her life that she stopped counting them and had learned at a young age that doctors didn't know how to care for her injuries, so she stopped seeking care for them.

Over the next months, she fought with her husband's employer to get the life insurance benefit he had through his job, which she finally did get. It was awkward as she worked at the same employer, and they did not make it easy for her. We talked on the phone often, and she came to the office for appointments a few times also, and as she worked through her grief, she formulated a plan for her life going forward. Despite her frailty, she planned to travel around the country, visiting friends, looking for somewhere to settle. Although she was fiercely independent, she had depended on Jim to help her with many daily activities, and now she was ready to reinvent her life, to truly begin anew. This plan entailed complex planning, as she was not able to board a plane on her own, so had to pay a companion to carry her aboard.

I heard from her from time to time, by phone and postcards from all over, then she called to tell me her final plans. She was going to relocate to another country, where she had a good friend, had bought a smallish farm, sight unseen, outside a small town, and she was excited to begin this new chapter. She had identified someone to travel with her, buying him a round-trip ticket for the help. She had already bought a specially equipped van, like the one she had here, that would be at the airport when she arrived. Once there, she busied herself getting to know her neighbors, who rented her land to graze their sheep, and she enlisted the children to help her with tasks, especially the young girls, who by custom, were expected to marry young, and not finish high school, to not even think about a career.

She was determined to change that. She bought two dogs, who she called her "fur kids", and we began a wonderful, year-long written correspondence. She was brilliant, had started her working life in technology, at IBM, and loved to tell me about how she had to make "the boys" see her point of view. This was an experience we shared, and it deepened our connection. Each letter I received in her distinctive handwriting, written with a fountain pen and on full sized lined white paper, was a treasure. She wrote candidly of her childhood, which was marred by a suspicion that her parents were abusing her, due to her many fractures, which led to her being removed from their custody by Child Protective Services, and to her being an only child. She mused about how this had shaped her personality and her relationship with her parents.

She was an amazing person, a very special friend and still many years later, I marvel at how she was able to begin again after Jim died. Sadly, she died several years ago, which is another story. I have all her letters, and so many years later, I marvel at her life force.

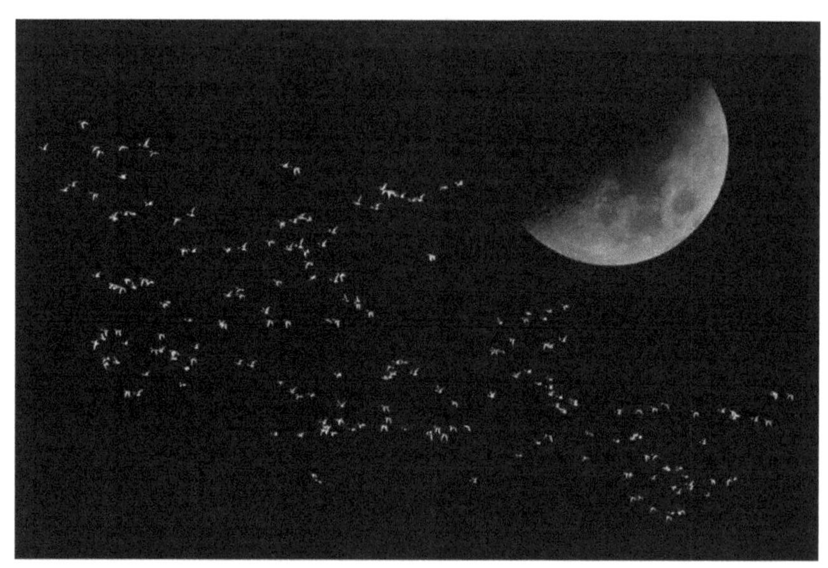

Night Flight - photograph by David C. Hurwitz, MD

The Power of Faith

By Bradley J. Winston, MD

I was brought up in a largely agnostic family whose major passion and commitment was progressive politics. In the terminology of the time, my mother, the daughter of Jewish immigrants from pogroms in the Ukraine and Russia, was a "red diaper" baby who was sent to Jewish socialist summer camps in upstate New York. My grandparents were tirelessly committed to the working people and the labor movement in New York.

My father, the son of a butcher, had parents who were Jewish Hungarian immigrants. He loved to share stories of how he carried a hundred pounds of beef on his back through many feet of snow to simply help make enough money to put himself through school. He was raised around Boston in an observant kosher Jewish household and eventually moved to New York to attend medical school. He met and married my mother, abandoned his kosher and religious upbringing, became committed to progressive politics, and favored what he referred to as a scientific and empiric world view. He was passionate about caring for those who could not care for themselves, not to achieve an exalted afterlife but because what we did now for those in need was the reward we could and should expect.

Indeed, it was his wish that his body be donated to an anatomy class. I must confess, the family never did carry out this wish and he was interred in a Jewish cemetery.

It was in the context of this world view that my parents raised their four children. We were always made aware of our Jewish heritage and identity. My parents refused to buy anything German, out of respect for those murdered in the Holocaust. My grandparents and parents spoke Yiddish and attended the Yiddish theatre but did not attend services at a synagogue. We were always reminded of what my parents felt was the core value of Judaism, to put others above ourselves and to help those who were less fortunate. While we were not members of a synagogue, we did celebrate the major Jewish holidays, but also a nonreligious Christmas, at which time my mother draped lights over our rubber tree which we referred to as the Chanukah bush. Thirteenth birthdays were singled out as unique and called a Bar Mitzvah, but we never recited from the Torah and did not attend temple services. Jehovah/Yahweh was a word we knew but not a concept that was part of our ingrained consciousness. We were deeply steeped in the culture, history, identity, and values of being Jewish but never in specific religious beliefs.

With this background I entered medical school where all of us at a much younger age than most of our nonmedical peer group were exposed to pain, disease, death and, ultimately also to the power of healing. The stress of this exposure to morbidity and mortality led many of us to think that joint pain meant we had lupus, our chest pain indicated cardiac disease. Fortunately, with time and experience, these anxieties abated, and we developed the ability to recognize that it was not us but the patient who had the disease, as Samuel Shem so insightfully observed in his satirical novel about medical interns appropriately entitled *The House of God.*

When I finally emerged as a practicing Gastroenterologist/Hepatologist, I became enamored of procedures and the ability to diagnose, treat, and help so many patients. Then, in my first year of practice, I encountered an extraordinary, engaging, and gracious fifty-five-year-old woman who presented to my clinic with difficulty swallowing, a terrible cough and weight loss. We diagnosed her with an esophageal cancer that eroded into her trachea. The next five months consisted of a brutal course of treatment involving esophageal stenting, surgery, radiation, and chemotherapy. During those five months we had become quite close. She had few family members, but I learned that the members of her church were her primary family and that her church and her faith were the most prominent and important parts of her life. Not one day in the hospital passed without her being attended to by fellow church members or her pastor.

As her condition continued to worsen, I became increasingly distressed when it became evident that she was likely to die. There was nothing else we could do to save her. We could only ameliorate her suffering with narcotics and respiratory support. Astonishingly, she often consoled me, noticing my own distress at her suffering and our inability to do more. She profoundly believed she was going to a better world where she would become one with God. Despite all our interventions, she continued to deteriorate and five months after the diagnosis she died. She retained her serenity and sense of peace to her last dying breath.

As time has passed, I have been blessed with the ability to help many people and the humility to accept that there are others we cannot help or save despite all our technology, knowledge, and best intentions. Over all of these years of practice and life, while I treasure my Jewish identity, I still have not joined a synagogue. Certainly, as time passes, I recognize that we have far more yesterdays than tomorrows and that mortality is inevitable. It is appealing on some level to believe that we might enter another life after this life. I have not ruled out the potential existence of a higher being. I do often think back to my strongly faith-based patient.

What I did learn so profoundly from this special individual, who comforted me during her dying moments in my first year of practice, is that the power of faith does have the ability to sustain those who do believe and to bring them peace even in the face of pain, suffering and inevitable mortality. Whether we share or do not share that faith, we certainly cannot deny its power.

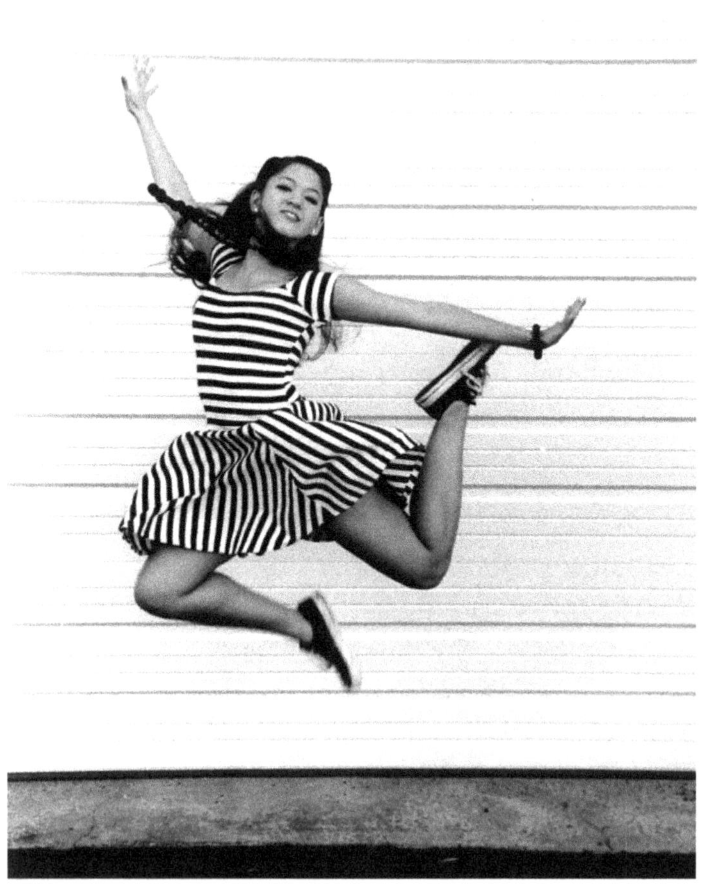

The Joy of Dancing - photograph by LoAn Nguyen, MD

The Contest

By Susan Boiko, MD

I was a sad, bedraggled pediatric intern, so depressed that I would frequently burst into tears for no reason. While rotating on Ward 8E, Cindy, a particularly annoying fourteen-year-old inpatient, would ride alongside me every morning in her motorized wheelchair as I made rounds, calling out in a loud voice for all to hear, "Susan, you're crying! Why are you crying?"

"It's just allergies, I'm not crying" I mumbled, trying to swat her away with a wave of my weary hand. That Saturday morning I'd been up all night, and Cindy, a lifelong resident of Ward 8E, was keenly aware of the comings and goings in her bailiwick. She had no problem poking her smart nose into my exhausted business. Born with osteogenesis imperfecta, she could not thrive outside the hospital, so she lived at the far end of the ward, in a private room that child life staff had made homey with a dresser, curtains, and a patchwork quilt on her hospital bed. An outstanding hospital-schooled student, with a teen-sized head perched precariously on a toddler-sized body, she knew every staff member and was the unofficial greeter for every admitted child.

That morning I had one final note to write before I could go home. I had admitted Shane, a fourteen-year-old boy from the Emergency Department, the night before at eight in the evening. I'd found him hunched over in the "asthma room," vomiting the pineapple juice he'd been given in a failed attempt to hydrate him. Wheezing noisily, he sat slumped in the wheelchair as I pushed him to his bed in an eight-bed ward and started his IV. Now it was eight on Saturday morning and I had waved off Cindy, hurrying to listen to Shane's lungs one last time and then to write a quick note, longing for my own bed.

But where was Shane? Not in his bed. None of the other patients had seen him. According to the nurse and ward clerk, "he was here a minute ago." Angry now, I worked my way through every room and bathroom. No Shane. As I got closer to the last room in the hall, Cindy's room, I could hear faint rock and roll music. I flung open the door to her room. There before me was an astonishing tableau. Shane stood in the corner, nodding his head to the beat, intently observing the actions of two teenaged girls in the room. Casually holding on to his IV pole with one hand, clad in back-to-back hospital gowns, I saw for the first time that he was six feet tall and handsome. Cindy was writhing and gesticulating in her wheelchair, head bobbing in time to the music. Elaine, another "frequent flyer" teen whose paraplegia from spina bifida surgery caused ulcers that required her to rest, stomach-down, on a too short "banana cart" was waving her arms in swimming motions with a big smile on her face.

My fried brain couldn't process it. "What's going on here?" I shouted. He motioned me a little closer, then whispered in my ear—"Sshh! It's a dance contest, and I'm the judge. Come back later."

Apologetically, I backed out of the room and closed the door softly. The past months had been a barrage of sick children, children who had been beaten, who had survived horrific car crashes, children who were allergic to cockroaches and were burned out of apartment after apartment. There were children whose parents drank liquor in the waiting area and threw the glass bottles on the floor, where I would try and scoop up the glass fragments as they dozed. For the first time I had seen a glimmer of normalcy in the lives of kids, one of whom lived in a hospital.

I didn't cry when I made rounds the next day, Cindy at my side. Instead, I told her she was a great dancer and that I'd bring her some of my old records from my parents' house.

Last Dance

By Carrie A. Horwitch MD,

M r. C. loved to do ballroom dancing. Perhaps that is why he chose me as his primary care doctor.

I met Mr. C. after he moved from Southern California to Seattle, to be closer to his daughter.

He was five-feet-ten, overly nourished with a receding hairline and a big smile.

After we chatted about the best places to find swing and lindy dancing, I tried to get him interested in looking into Cajun/Zydeco dancing. After the initial discussion about dancing, he expressed the main reason for his visit.

"I just feel like I can't get enough air into my lungs"- worry flitted across his face.

"My docs in California, couldn't find anything wrong and told me to lose weight. I'm not sure I believe them."

His exam that day did not reveal any abnormality that would explain his symptoms. I was puzzled.

I arranged for him to see me in a couple of months, after I could review his prior health records, to determine if further testing was warranted.

His medical records arrived. They made the book *War and Peace* look small. His doctors had done an extensive workup - heart, lungs, sleep study and more - without a specific abnormality found. I would be frustrated also.

When Mr. C. returned to the clinic - I was hoping his symptoms had improved.

"No, Doc, just the same as before. I even notice it at night now when I lie down to sleep."

This time his exam showed a subtle difference in the movement of his chest. One side did not move as well as the other. Chest x-rays confirmed my suspicion.

Aha, I thought - the large muscle at the bottom of the chest - the diaphragm has a problem.

I confidently told Mr. C. - "your diaphragm is partially frozen - I think that is the cause of your symptoms. We'll have you see neurology for more testing and workup."

The diagnosis was much worse than anticipated. It was not a partially paralyzed diaphragm.

Mr. C. had ALS - amyotrophic lateral sclerosis/ Lou Gehrig's disease.

This is a progressive neuromuscular condition for which there was no good treatment or cure. The muscle function would continue to deteriorate and eventually lead to loss of body functions-walking, bowel control, eating and breathing- all the while the mind stays alert. It is a fatal diagnosis.

The next time I saw Mr. C. his attitude was positive.

"Look, Doc, as long as I can still do my dancing, I'll be satisfied." He spoke with a tone that hinted he felt otherwise.

Our visits became more about his goals of care and quality of life. He was adamant he would not want any breathing tubes or interventions to prolong his life. He valued body function over length of life.

We met several times over the months each time he renewed his end of life wishes. He assured me he had discussed his end-of-life care with his daughter-his surrogate decision maker.

On what would be our last clinic visit-he struggled to walk the hallway. Moving at a snail's pace - the effort making him sweat.

He realized ALS was robbing him of his movements. He asked me for one thing that day.

Would I please do a Lindy swing dance with him?

I hesitated briefly - is it ethically OK to dance with my patient?

Sure, I said a moment later

One, two, three, four, five, six, seven, eight - even with a twirl at the end. We did the Lindy step right there in my office.

He smiled as he left my office - his steps a little quicker than when he had arrived.

Several weeks later I was called STAT to the emergency room.

Mr. C. was lying on the bed, shallow breaths, his lips looking like he ate a bowl of blueberries. His daughter, whom I had never met, looked scared and upset.

"Do something, he can't breathe," she cried frantically.

I took Mr. C.'s hand (now cold from lack of oxygen) thankfully he was still conscious.

"Can you hear me, Mr. C.?" - a quick nod yes

"Do you want us to put you on a breathing machine?" an emphatic shake of the head, NO!

I asked him again more for his daughter's sake than my own. "Mr. C., your breathing is very bad, and we need to act now if you want to be intubated and help you breathe. Again, his head shake confirmed NO.

The daughter's anger turned to grief as tears streamed down her face like a faucet.

I squeezed Mr. C.'s hand and assured him that we would keep him comfortable and respect his wishes.

I thanked him for the privilege of being his doctor and for the honor of having had the "Last Dance".

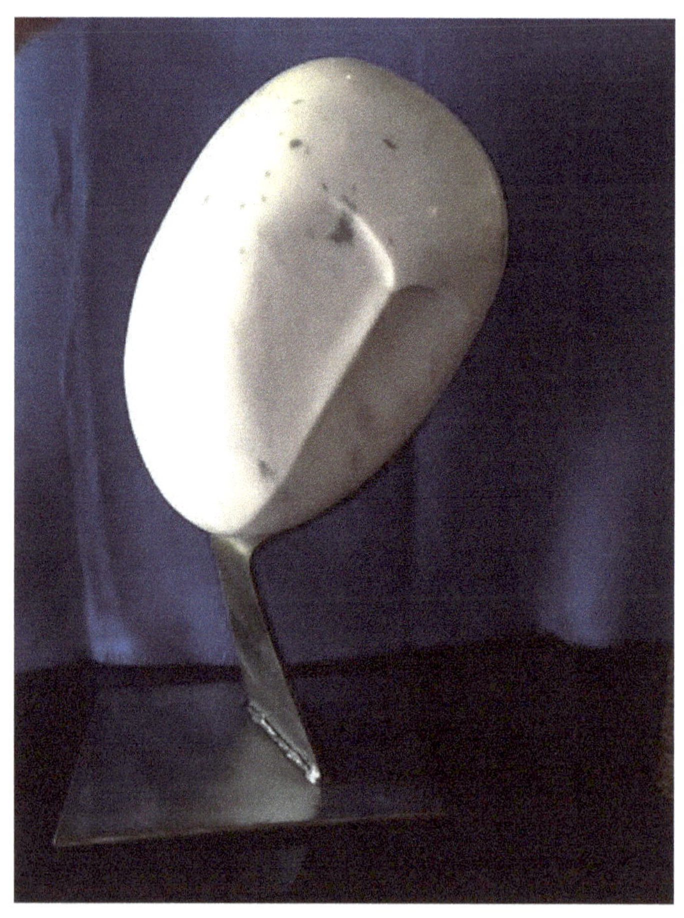

Contemplation - marble by Kenneth Elconin, MD

The Beauty of a Crooked Smile

By Scott Abramson, MD

Maria works as an aide in a nursing home. She spends many hours changing the diapers of lots of old and sick folks. I saw her in the neurology clinic because the right side of her face had become paralyzed, a condition we call Bell's Palsy. When I saw her, it was one month after the paralysis began, and the right side of her face was still partly paralyzed. Though the paralysis usually gets better with time, Maria was worried it might not. But she was worried for a different reason than most. "Doctor Abramson," she confided, "I'm afraid I won't get my smile back. And sometimes, Doctor, for my patients, all I have to give... is a smile."

Those were her words.

Let me repeat them:

"Sometimes for my patients, Doctor, all I have to give... is a smile."

(And we are talking about giving a smile to sick, old folks who probably can't even remember her name.)

If I were in Maria's place, and my face was paralyzed and disfigured, I can guarantee you, those would not be my words.

Yet I cannot help but have this thought:

When I meet folks like Maria, I am humbled by their beauty.

I am humbled by their beauty, no matter how crooked the smile.

CHAPTER FOUR
Pandemic Pause

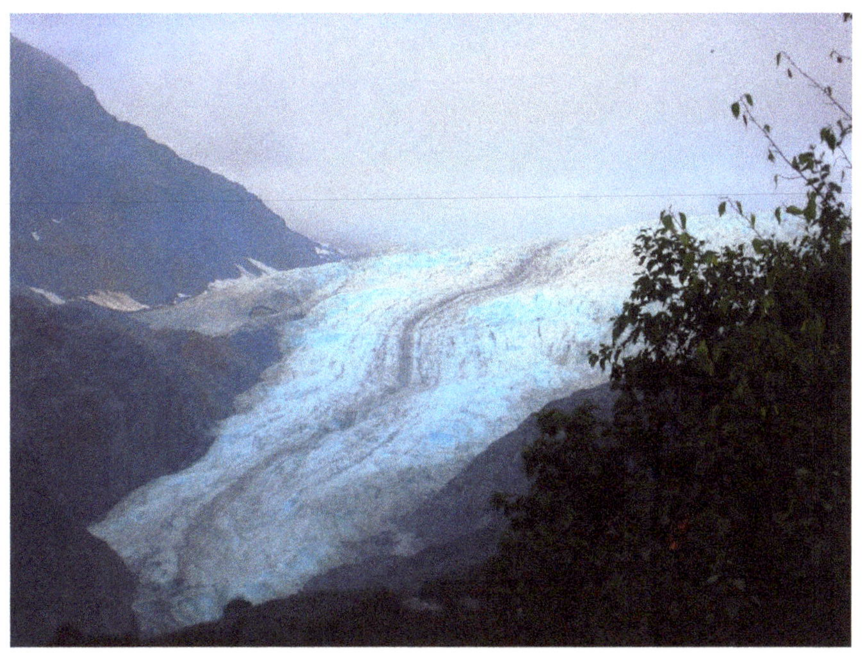

Alaska's Exit Creek - photograph by Craig Sadur, MD

The Irony of Joy in a Pandemic

By Tom E. Norris, MD

To find joy in the middle of a pandemic.
An exercise that's strangely academic.
And yet I find I'm feeling glad
For recent blessings I have had.

Good health for me and my family,
We've had through steps followed cannily.
Yes washing, yes masking, and distancing too.
We kept out Covid and even the flu.

But the biggest joy we've recently seen—
Came from a small jab of good vaccine.
The doors and windows opened a bit,
The path ahead more brightly lit.

The joy was dimmed when we all felt a—
Steady approach of the deadly Delta.
But even that strain's beginning to fade.
We can move ahead with plans long made.

To find some joy when surrounded by pain,
Seems strange to some but fits my brain.
We must rejoice over little things.
We are still here! What will the future bring?

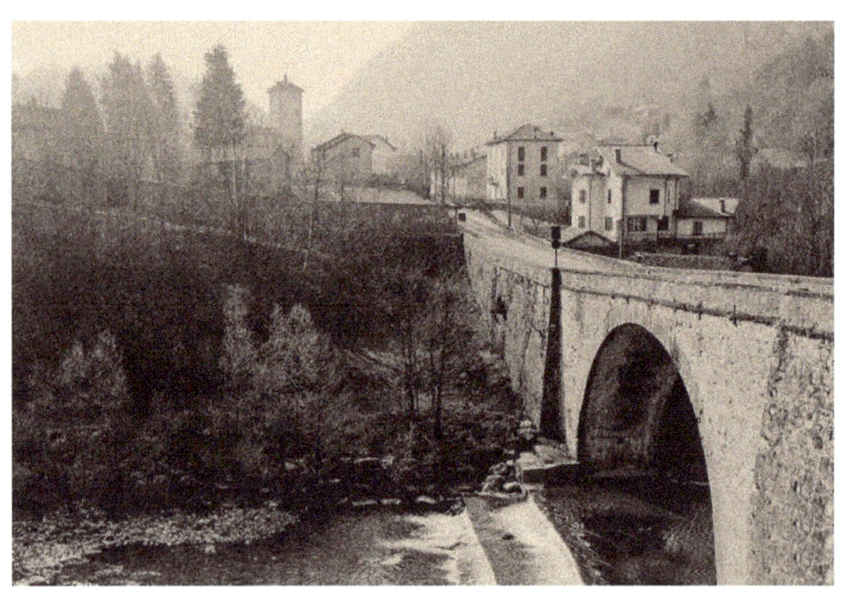

Voltaggio Italy - photograph by David C. Hurwitz, MD

Medical Histories Recall The 1918 Spanish Flu Pandemic

By Henry W. Eisenberg, MD

In the time of Covid, enduring lockdowns and isolation, I often thought of a small group of patients whom I treated from 1975 to 1985. At that time, I was a young GI surgeon in private practice. While taking the medical history prior to the use of electronic medical records, and asking about medications, my patient, age seventy-five and female, told me that she takes Castor oil every day because "it SAVED ME from the Spanish Flu." After this initial patient, I heard similar stories from seven more women. All were in their seventies and early eighties and all survived 1918 pandemic and continued taking daily Castor oil. They lived long, healthy lives, part of the "greatest generation" spanning the Depression and World War II. Some were teachers. One had been a golf champion; most were active participants in community activities. All were proud of their children. I clearly remember one of these patients, Mrs. W. She had two sons: one was the U.S. Ambassador to Austria and her other son was a psychiatrist in California. Of course, she told me all about "my son the doctor." Perhaps she assumed I knew all about the Ambassador. But we know where her maternal pride glowed the brightest.

Back forty years ago, I never imagined living through such a devastating pandemic. My initial impression of these Castor oil histories was one of skepticism. It seemed like folklore, unscientific. There were no trials, no controls. Was I hearing old wives' tales? Was this an early version of an American President advocating for chloroquine to cure Covid? Of course, available therapy in 1918 was limited. In the absence of antibiotics, antivirals, and vaccines, over the counter remedies were widely used. Documented 1918 treatments were: aspirin, quinine, ammonia, turpentine, salt water, decongestants. Laxatives such as Castor oil were available in most homes and were thought to expel toxins. Sound familiar? There was not much doctors could do. No respirators. The news of the day was dominated by War and Peace. Many more people died of the Flu than the guns of World War I.

Intrigued by what my patients told me so many years ago, I was inspired to take a deeper dive into medical holistic, and naturopathic literature. Castor oil is a thick, odorless oil made from seeds of the castor plant, Ricinus communis. Its biologically active ingredient is Ricinoleic acid, which has been shown to activate intestinal smooth muscle. Castor oil is an important component for soaps and cosmetics. Claims for Castor oil medicinal and beauty benefits date to Cleopatra. Such a lineage may explain its mystique. Among the most widely recognized indications and claims for castor oil are: 1) Enhanced immunity. 2) Effective laxative. 3) Skin treatments. 4) Obstetric applications. 5) Emollient for enlarged lymph nodes. 6) Topical for arthritis and back pain.

Such a wide range of potential benefits or this medicinal oil may explain my patients' loyalty and enthusiasm. But alas, there are adverse events associated with chronic castor oil ingestion: gastrointestinal cramps, abdominal pain, irregular bowel function with both constipation and diarrhea

In the late 1970s, these side effects led to this special cohort of patients being referred to gastrointestinal specialists. When we evaluated them looking into their stomachs and intestines, we only found minor changes usually related to laxatives. The technical term is "cathartic colon." Ultimately this led to the formulation of newer laxatives with a different mode of action.

We are left to wonder. What medications will future generations associate with the 2020 Covid pandemic? Will mRNA technology lead to cancer therapies? Will the anti-vaxxers be ridiculed or lead to more anti-science beliefs? Will we live to see more pandemics? My more lasting lesson would be to listen to our patients, think about what they say, and learn.

History in the Making: A Case of Community Transmission

By Betsy Strong, MD

In December 2019, we started hearing of a mysterious flu-like illness causing severe disease and death in Wuhan, China. By mid-January 2020, the full genome of the virus causing the illness had been sequenced by a Chinese scientist and shared with international scientists. By late January, cases of the same illness were appearing in other countries in Asia, in Europe, and in the U.S. By February, the virus was labeled SARS-CoV-2 and the illness COVID-19.

In February 2020, the Centers for Disease Control and Prevention (CDC) developed a PCR test for the detection of SARS-CoV-2 in clinical specimens. The tests were in short supply. To qualify for the test, the person suspected of having the illness had to have: 1) symptoms of COVID-19 and a history of recent travel to Wuhan, China; or 2) symptoms of and known exposure to COVID-19. The local county Public Health Department (PHD) needed assistance of a locum physician to manage the deluge of test inquiries and authorization of sample collection. I signed up, answering after hours COVID-19-related calls from local urgent care clinics and emergency departments, rotating call with the Public Health Department officers. Due to a recent embargo on travel from China, the call was relatively quiet at first. If a patient met the strict criteria for the test, we would call Atlanta, speak with the CDC officer, present the history, and obtain a code. This code would then be attached to the clinical specimen. The specimen would be sent to the local Public Health Department, then forwarded to CDC, the test turnaround time was up to six or seven days.

On February 26th, a friend and former colleague of mine was asked to provide an infectious disease consultation at the local community hospital. The patient was a sixty-five-year-old woman who had been admitted six days prior for a severe respiratory illness and she was not improving. She did not have any known risk factors for COVID-19: she lived at home with an elderly mother who had mild respiratory symptoms; neither of them had traveled out of the Bay Area nor had a known exposure. As my colleague reviewed the record, she thought "Could this be COVID-19?" All other tests and cultures had been unremarkable, and the clinical scenario seemed consistent with a SARS-like illness.

Incidentally, my colleague had been sitting at the computer just outside the patient's room in the ICU. She was staring at images of the patient's chest CT, "it looked just like the images being published of patients in China with COVID-19." The ICU rooms were single patient rooms, separated from the common hallway without a door or divider. I relayed this story to my husband. A former hospitalist at that hospital - having sat in that spot for hours over the years - he immediately visualized it. He said he would have had a reaction like Frodo Baggins in the Lord-of-the-Rings scene where the world devolved into tunnel vision around him as he encountered the ring-wraiths on the road out of Hobbiton.

My colleague immediately placed the patient into airborne and contact isolation, informed the hospital Infection Prevention nurse, and reached out to the county PHD to obtain permission to test the patient. She was told, as expected, that this patient did not qualify for testing. However, a news alert had just been released that afternoon, describing the first case of community-acquired COVID-19 in the U.S. - in nearby Solano County. Though it was now seven o'clock in the evening, my colleague reached out again to the PHD. She made a strong case to the covering officer and got permission. The specimen was immediately collected from the patient and sent to the county PHD the next day. That day was the first day the PHD lab was able to process its own PCR test, allowing a rapid test turnaround in twenty-four hours. My colleague got a call the next day that the test was positive! It meant that this Santa Clara County case was the second known case of community transmission of COVID-19 in the U.S.

Overnight, the CDC protocol for testing changed: now travel to Wuhan China or a history of exposure was no longer required for testing. Nationwide, case counts for COVID-19 shot up. More embargoes were placed on international travel. At clinics and hospitals, protocols for personal protective equipment and isolation were set up. PCR testing became more widely available. Masking became mandated. Social distancing and other measures were encouraged. COVID-19 was declared a pandemic by the World Health Organization (WHO) on March 11. A shelter in place - the first of its kind in the country - was ordered by the Santa Clara County PHD Director on March 16.

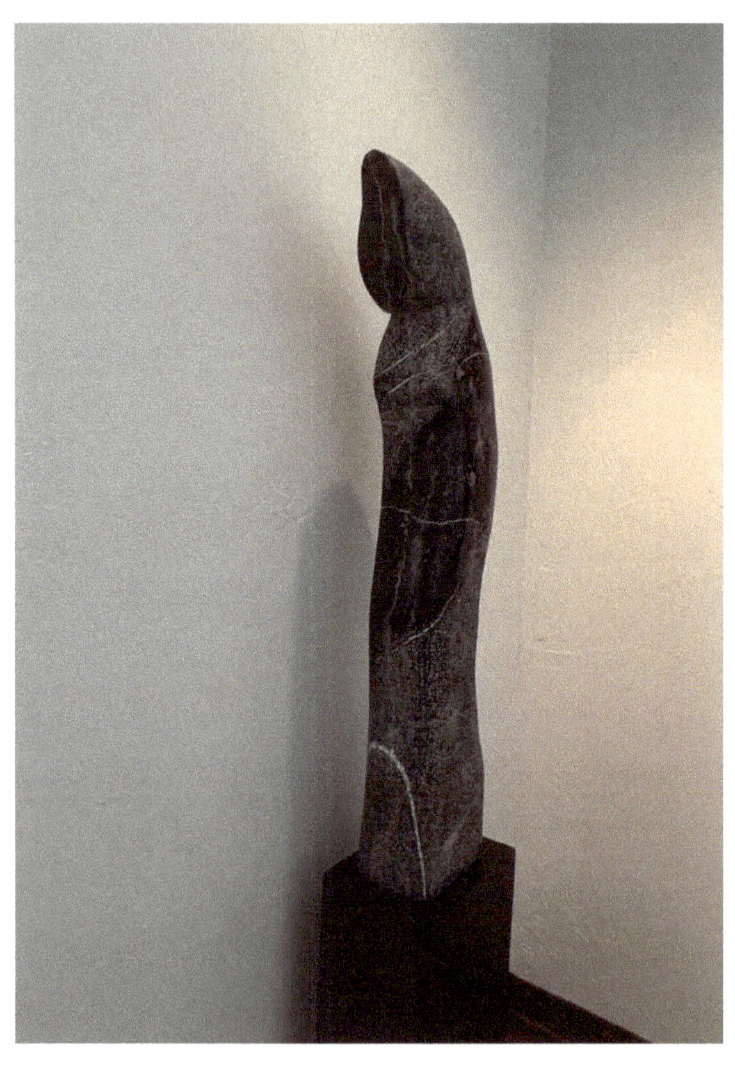

Hooded Woman - marble by Kenneth Elconin, MD

"It's nothing"

By David P. Hurwitz, MD

Sweet aromas fading, coffee tasting awful
Each step heavy, a trudging pace
A hint of scratchiness

"It's nothing" so some say

Coldness descends, an oscillating quiver
Inner kindling now a flame, trying to fend off the unseen
Engulfed, losing bearings, the barrage continues

Now a simmer, a brief respite
Emerging from my cocoon, I still recognize me, my room
I shakily arise, dizzy, vision sketchy
Brace myself against the nightstand, taking several cool sips
Trying to recharge for the next round

"It's nothing" so some say

Back and forth we tango, my reserves thin
My nemesis ramps it up

The cough erupts, dry and furious
Long rhythmic spasms, ribs sore and tired
Conversation cut mid-sentence,
little time for an uninterrupted breath
Cough syrup useless

Breathing quickens and shortens
Attempts at deep breathing are further dampened by a new,
intensely dagger like pain mid back
The fusillade continues. I lose consciousness

"It's nothing" so some say

I awaken some days later, sustained by machines
Nurse and staff shuttle in and out
Medication infused, utility unknown,
a mad scramble to defang the beast
My beloved is at my side, anxious, tearful

I am oddly relieved, no longer fighting solo
Each day I strengthen, breathe more forcefully
The machines drop from the scene
I slowly reboot, back to me

Guilt and Gratitude

By Prasad Palakurthy, MD

The alarming WhatsApp messages started coming in as my four-year-old and six-year-old grandchildren played on the floor of our Lafayette, California home. It was March 11, 2020, and since moving a year ago to California, it had quickly become a new favorite ritual for my grandkids to stay with us on Friday evenings. The messages arrived on a medical school classmate's WhatsApp group: "World Health Organization has declared a pandemic." "CDC director has said the pandemic will get much worse." "The National Basketball Association has canceled a game due to virus concerns." As the messages kept pouring in from my classmates, feelings of gratitude began to co-evolve with a gnawing sense of guilt; feelings that would only deepen as this long pandemic has worn on.

Guilt and gratitude are two human emotions from opposite spectrums. The majority of times a particular situation in our life may bring out one of the two emotions but rarely both emotions together. From our childhood we are taught to "count our blessings." This is emphasizing the positive feeling of gratitude. Feeling guilty is mostly discouraged. However, sometimes these opposite feelings co-exist.

The pandemic has had a myriad of impacts on different people. On the one hand, people who are infected with the virus have suffered tremendously including the ultimate sacrifice of death. Workers in the hospitality industry and manual labor suffered quite a bit, including greater exposure risk to Covid, a loss of jobs, and all the subsequent consequences of losing those jobs. On the other hand, people on the high end of the socioeconomic spectrum - those with a good education, tech jobs, etc. - have been able to continue their jobs, often from home, without any financial loss. In fact, many even found their net worth increasing as they saved money with less travel, less dining out, and a massive uptick in the stock market. As a retired physician living within miles of my children and grandchildren, I have experienced my own Covid contradictions in the two intense reactions the pandemic has elicited in me as a retired physician and grandparent: guilt and gratitude.

I was a practicing cardiologist in Des Moines, Iowa for thirty-two years. In December of 2018, I decided to retire and move to the San Francisco Bay Area, as our three children settled in the area. Still, I missed practicing medicine and looked for ways to continue. Although I worked as a locum physician in 2019, I worked mostly as a volunteer physician at a local free clinic, Rotacare Clinic. With the onset of Covid all onsite clinics were closed, and only virtual visits were open. As my colleagues and friends were in the trenches and facing the battle of Covid, I felt intense guilt remaining at my home without facing any risk. To decrease my guilt, I tried to sign up for a list of retired physicians who could be called in case of need.

At the same time, though, I also felt intense gratitude. Because we had moved to the Bay Area before the pandemic, we were able to spend a significant amount of time with our children and grandchildren. Even at the worst of the Covid infections, we were able to see them as part of the same bubble. Instead of seeing them through a screen, we saw them in the flesh. If I were still practicing in the Midwest, that would not have been possible.

As retired physicians, we want to contribute to the benefit of society. We have expertise that we've built up over decades, but often lack opportunities to give back our expertise short of full-time practice. In this regard, organizations like MAVEN Project are contributing to fill the void. I wish there were more organizations like that.

At the end of two years of pandemic we are frequently caught between these two diverse human emotions. We hope and pray that we are done with the pandemic.

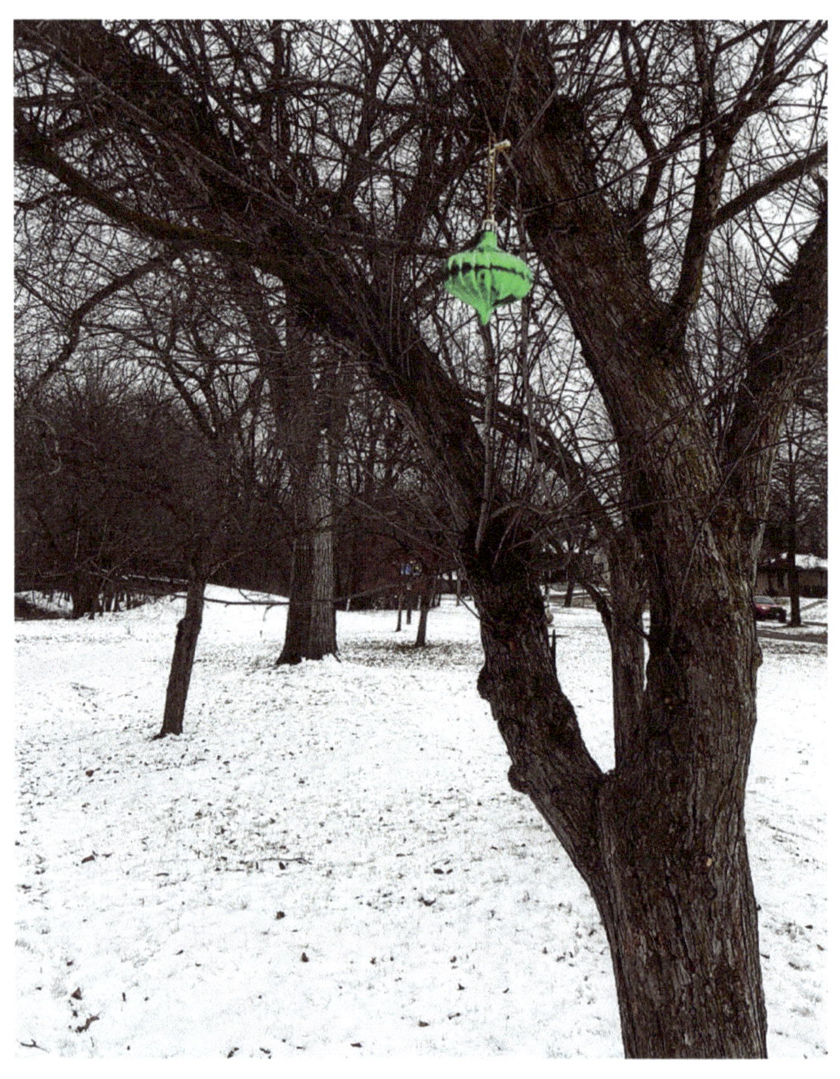

A Bright Spot - photograph by Cynthia C. Leigh, MD

Joy

By Lois Freedman, MD

Joy, something hard to experience during these pandemic times. For myself as a geriatric psychiatrist I think I have gained a deeper understanding of the meaning of anhedonia.

In mid-March 2020 while I was headed to visit my ninety-six-year-old mom in her nursing facility my husband called to inform me that this might be our last in person visit as nursing facilities were locking down.

Joy experienced in very brief bursts - getting through to the nurse's station on the phone once a week, if we were lucky, FaceTime calls from the facility so I could see my mom's smile.

And then came the call that she had Covid. With consultations from MAVEN Project colleagues and medical school roommate, a public health MD, I was able to advocate for appropriate treatment – small joys.

My mom recovered and then joy became weekly outdoor visits with masking and hearing challenges to deal with.

In the fall my mom was able to fill out her absentee ballot – she never missed an election – true joy.

My mom died on December 24, 2020, at the age of ninety-seven. She was a woman full of joy raised in a challenging world who died in a challenging time.

I treasure every phone and FaceTime call I had with her in her final months – her smile was a thing of joy.

The Jab

by David P. Hurwitz, MD

Virion assembly lines ramp up production, genomes mix, deadlier versions emerge
The unseen foe collects more bodies, seemingly unopposed

Masks help, but more is needed. The jab arrives!

First came the health care workers, jab…jab…jab
Then the vulnerable, elderly, frail, chronically ill, jab…jab
Then the rest of us…jab

Then came the skeptics
Some genuine in their concern
The jab was created "too fast", the technology "too new", too many unknowns

Others more hardened in their views, anti-vaxxers, those beholden to "Freedom"
Some simply vulnerable, easily misled, misdirected

Fed by massive weaponized propaganda machines, social media, TV networks, a freakish Messiah
Money making misinformation amplified at scale

Outrage, anger, Yes or No, Us versus Them, For or Against…
Vaccines laden with tracking devices, 4G, now 5G, a miracle of modern engineering!

Hundreds of millions of arms jabbed, not one Zombie results!
The jabs stall, more are sickened
A new brew stirs, Delta hatches and pushes back at scale

The monster cares none for money, stature, politics, religion
Wanting only warm bodies to mass reproduce

The appeals widen, the mandates take hold
More start to "get it", some reluctantly acquiesce, others fight on, resist
Now at several billions of jabs with boosters on the way

Well off societies forge slowly toward normalcy, those less fortunate fight for first jabs
Always the same

As masks are shed, friends reunite but perhaps too soon as Omicron scales the globe
We are now used to this game, shrug a bit, endure, and witness as Omicron recedes into viral obscurity

When "normal" eventually returns what will we have learned?

Will fresh memories of despair and challenge dissipate into complacency, or will we harden our defenses against the next incursion?

Will we become a more "we" centric species, caring not just for ourselves and immediate circle, but for strangers both nearby and in distant lands? That perhaps is the best defense.

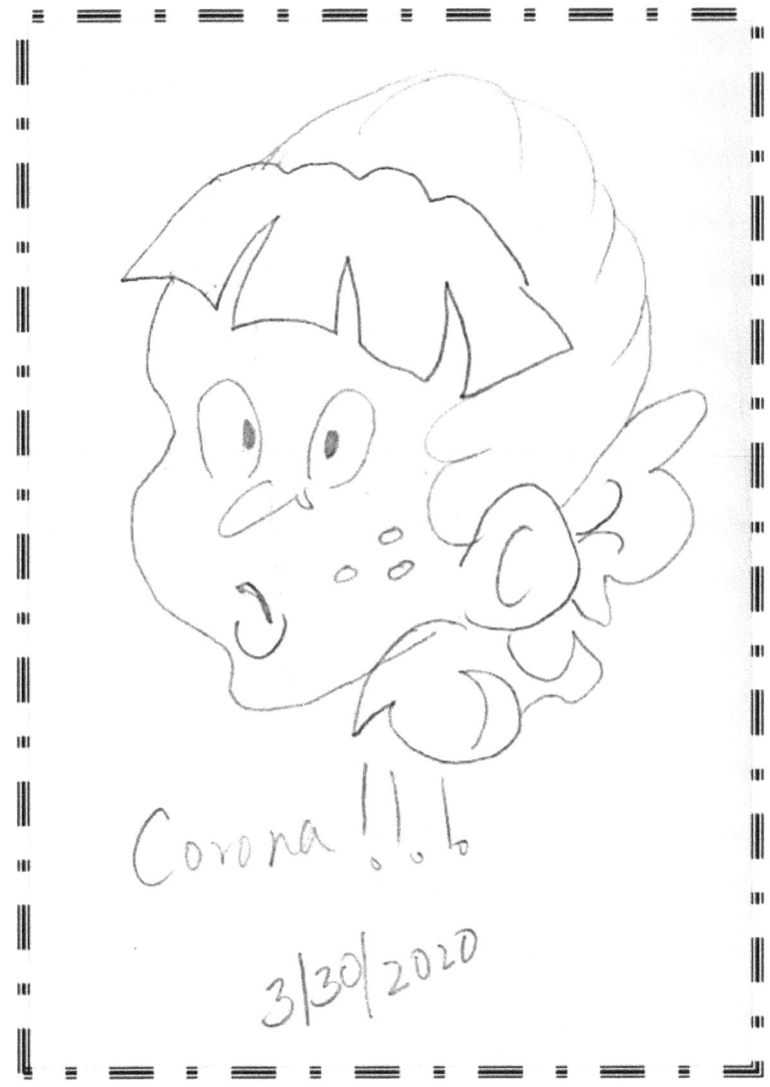

Corona - charcoal by Prasanna Menon, MD

Humanity & Resilience

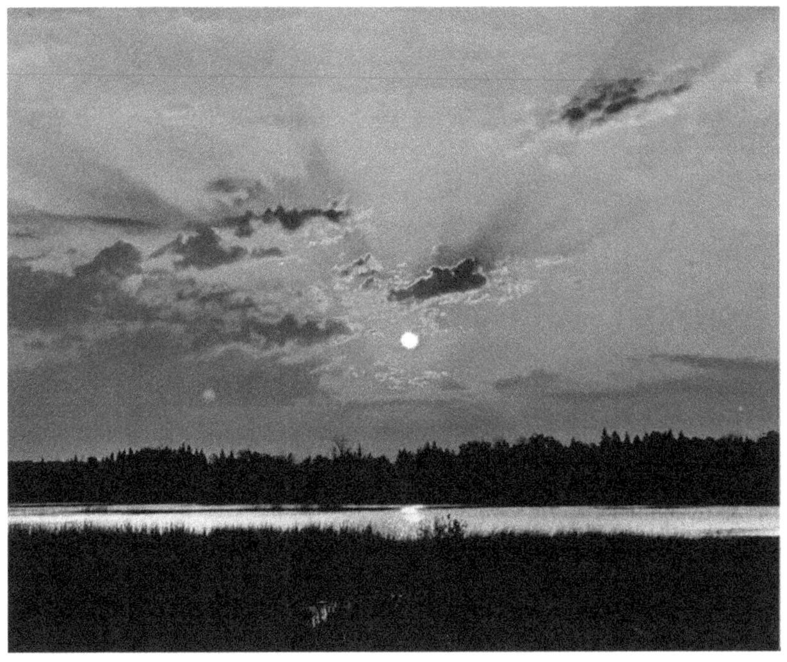

Moon Greets Sun - Kangaroo Lake - photograph by Barbara Loeb, MD

What Life Does

When we're not looking

By Barbara Loeb, MD

When we're stuck
telling ourselves
I'm not good enough
smart enough
attractive enough
resilient enough
or whatever enough.

When we see our children
becoming parents
and our parents turning away
as they leave this earth
and we realize more than half
our life is over
and we struggle because we've
lost our way.

That's when -- Life
taps us on the shoulder
and whispers "Hey you!"

That "Hey you" can appear
in many unexpected ways;
with grief
loss or sadness,
with celebration
joy or great happiness.

It can come
when we see the tiniest bud
peek through the melting snow,
smell the savory aroma
of cinnamon nuts roasting,
hear the hollow echoes
of rain drops on the pavement,
or feel the vibration
of cricket legs rubbing.

Life, in its unique way beckons:
"Hey you------you there!
Come sit beside me
under the magnolia tree."

Front Row Seat to Humanity

By Craig Sadur, MD

Years ago, we had the privilege of taking care of a very nice older gentleman, who suffered the ravages of diabetes. One event that he greatly anticipated was attending his granddaughter's upcoming wedding. Unfortunately, because of the progression of his peripheral arterial disease, he required urgent vascular surgical repair on his lower extremity. As fate would have it, his acute hospital stay included the date of the wedding. Understandably crestfallen, he was quite sad during that time, particularly while the wedding was taking place. The staff did their best to cheer him up but to no avail.

Then suddenly to everyone's great surprise and delight, the surgical ward elevator door opened. Out came his granddaughter resplendent in her wedding gown. Dedicated and loving to her grandfather, she had come directly from the ceremony to the hospital. His face lit up brightly while there was not one dry eye among the staff members.

One of the greatest honors of providing medical care is that we have a front row seat to humanity. We can repeatedly witness the finest aspects of people.

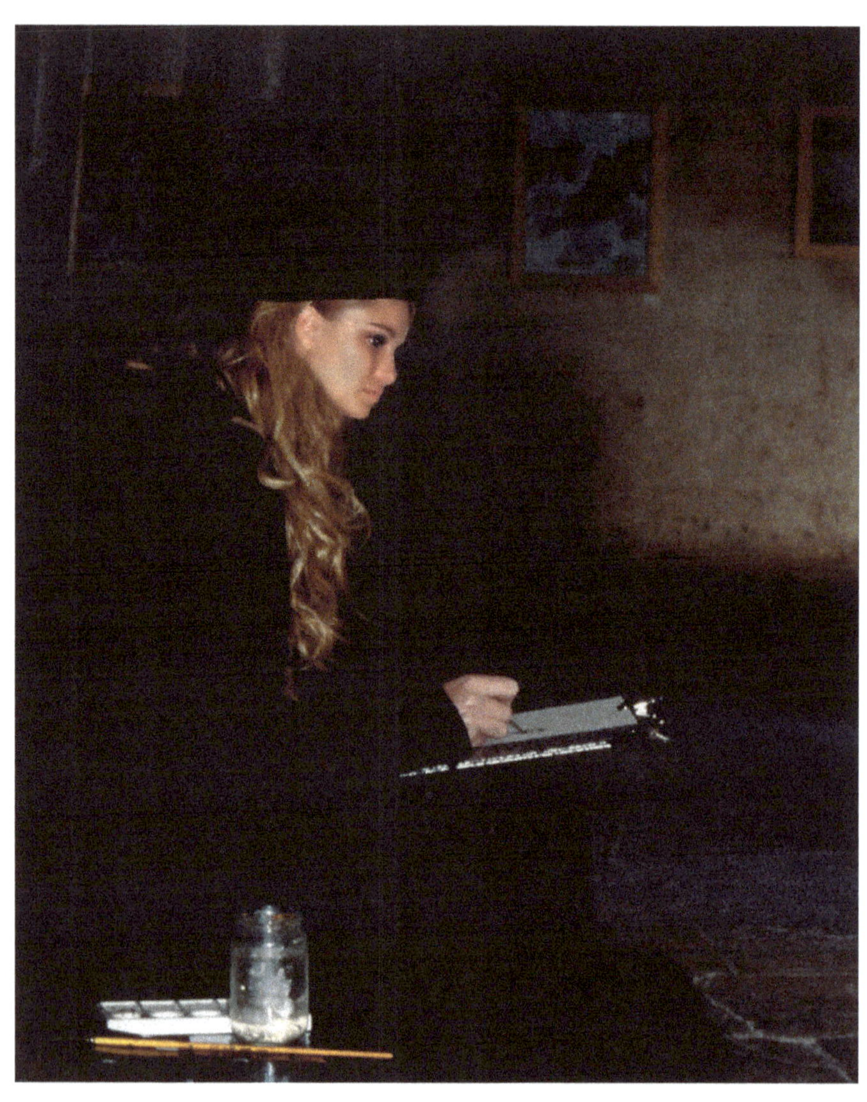

The Artist - photograph by David C. Hurwitz, MD

Resilience

By David C. Hurwitz, MD

I have often wondered where resilience comes from. Are we born with resilience? Or do we emerge, or not, after being tested? Certainly, the recent focus on PTSD would suggest that some of us are more resilient than others, and there may be a biochemical basis for this difference, but so far very little has been elucidated. Can one become more resilient? I suppose so. If you want to see resiliency in action and get a good laugh, watch the streaming series *Schitt's Creek*, where a formerly wealthy family has to start a new life in near poverty.

I don't have to look far to find resilience in my family. My wife Cindy has a wealth of it. In 1988, she was hit by a small bus while bicycling in Tahiti, breaking her tibia and four ribs. Treated with no significant pain medications, forced to ride in the back of a pickup truck, go by outrigger canoe across the Bora Bora lagoon, get loaded on an ancient De Haviland Otter airplane and flown to Papeete, Cindy complained of pain, but there wasn't a shred of self-pity. After a couple of days in a thirty-year-behind-the-times French hospital, we were flown home and she was hospitalized briefly to reset the fracture. It took nine months for her to get well, during which time she set about her physical therapy with a vengeance and few complaints. I've noticed the same pattern in her subsequent knee and hip replacements, the latter from which she is still having difficulty after seven months.

Cindy has also shown an emotional resilience far beyond my meagre abilities. My best Cindy story about resilience has to do with a particular client she had in her job as a travel agent. Kind and always patient, I think my wife would have made an excellent physician. One day she acquired a new client, whom we will call Jim. Jim was referred to by a neighbor who was a professor of psychology at a local university. Cindy found dealing with him to be problematic from their first encounter. Asking him where he wanted to go on his trip, he replied, "I don't know, uh Alaska, maybe Europe, the South Pacific, Africa, India, South America. Why don't you send me brochures on all of them?

"Jim," Cindy replied. "That's a lot of stuff to mail. Why don't we narrow it down?" He couldn't.

Over the years, every trip started like this. Every trip was a painful exercise in waiting for him to decide before it was too late to even go on the vacation. When he chose to remarry after two divorces, he couldn't decide where to go on his honeymoon. Even when Cindy begged him to make up his mind before we left on our upcoming trip, he couldn't do it, and finally with three days left before the marriage, one of Cindy's colleagues had to complete the travel plans. When he returned, Cindy discovered that he and his new wife were living in separate homes because they couldn't decide which one to move into together. Throughout her encounters with Jim, Cindy never lost her temper, always worked with him to get a trip planned, and used everything she had ever learned in obtaining her master's in educational psychology to cope with his indecisiveness.

Sometime later, Cindy happened to run into our neighbor and asked, "By the way, what does Jim do at the university?"

"Jim? Oh, he runs seminars in procrastination and decision-making," she replied.

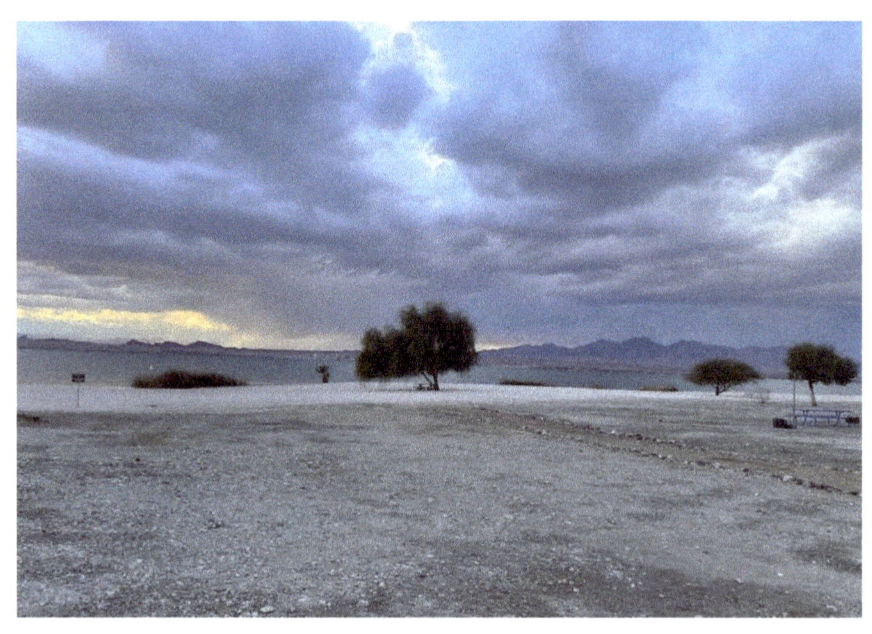

Out of Isolation - Lake Havasu - photograph by Barbara B. Loeb, MD

UN-BECOMING

By Richard Rapport, MD

I knew I wanted to go to medical school by the time I was ten years old. My thoracic surgeon father had introduced me to the local county hospital when I was five. I loved going there and watching the activity, while admittedly not fully understanding much, from that first day he stashed me in the nurses' station as he made rounds. My dad never suggested to me that I should become a doctor, but I wanted to be like him.

I prepared as an undergrad by taking a double major in biology and chemistry route offered at my liberal arts college to get us into med school. It worked, and I spent four of the happiest years of my life at the University of Michigan from 1965 to 1969. Believe me, even with the demands of a medical education, during those years it was impossible not to have fun in "The People's Republic of Ann Arbor."

While medical students see patients, examine them, take histories and so on, they don't really have much responsibility for them. That's what the intern year is about; learning to take responsibility for others. My internship seemed to me the most demanding year of my life, and was complicated by the Vietnam War, a "Sword of Damocles" dangling over every recently graduated physician at that moment. Everyone younger than thirty thought the war was a gigantic mistake, and it was.

In 1970, my choices for avoiding Vietnam were the Faustian bargain of the Berry Plan, Canada, jail, or the U.S. Public Health Service (USPHS), specifically National Institutes of Health (NIH). But lots of my contemporaries also wanted to spend two years doing research at NIH rather than treating trauma in SE Asia, so those jobs were hard to get. Somehow, I was selected. NIH not only protected me from the draft but also taught me valuable research skills. I thought I wanted to become an academic eventually as did many of my NIH contemporaries, so we all busily applied for residencies and headed toward a career. We began to become what we eventually were going to be. I certainly didn't see "my career" that way in the beginning, but I had started to become a neurosurgeon.

There were lots of steps on that path. Neurosurgical residency was of course a grueling and sometimes demeaning process of training. Even when you are learning to do things that are required by the specialty, sometimes out of necessity, you pretend that you already know how to do them. I did some reasonable research, got it published, went to meetings, met people, looked for work. After I finished my residency at University of Washington (UW), all the academic jobs I was offered were on the East Coast and in places my wife and I didn't want to live.

So, we left the country.

There was some money remaining in a grant from the China Medical Board sending UW specialists to the University of Malaya. Along with my fellow resident and close friend we both decided we'd become better surgeons and do more good in the world by going to teach at the University of Malaya in Kuala Lumpur than by staying put. We were there as the only fully trained neurosurgeons in the country for eighteen months and treated diseases we'd never heard about or even imagined. But as the time came to return, I still needed a job.

Fortunately, one was offered at what was then called Group Health Cooperative. This was appealing for a variety of reasons, and I accepted. For the next twenty-nine years I perfected my surgical abilities. During that time, I became a medical executive, a chief of various components, served on committees, involved myself in Seattle communities, and had a child. My wife began to publish books of magnificent short stories. We both became active in Seattle politics.

Nearing sixty-five, I wasn't the same technical surgeon I had been, and started to slow down. At that same moment, the Chairman of the Department of Neurosurgery at UW needed a senior person to help manage the huge service at Harborview. I became a clinical professor, an advisor to the residents, a listener and teacher for medical students, a resource for ICU nurses, a senior figure with enough gravitas to be believable. I again served on committees, went to meetings, saw families, made rounds, lectured, put out fires.

Then I retired and it all ended. Like many goal-directed people, I was very successful at becoming. I have now started to learn how to un-become, which is harder.

I still wake up at five-thirty in the morning, make my wife coffee, eat a small breakfast, look at my two email accounts and the news. Then, what?

The pace of daily life has diminished to a walk. I used to catch the bus at a corner near my house that took me directly to the front door of the Ninth and Jefferson office building at Harborview in fifteen minutes. I drive by that corner now with a sense of longing to again be the first one getting on, greet the driver, complain about Trump, and settle into the seat near the back door on the higher level behind an odd partition separating that seat from those getting off. The majority of the people who rode that Number Three bus in the morning work in hospitals or clinics on pill hill, and many know one another. Therefore, real conversations occurred between seat mates and across the aisles instead of hunched faces staring fixedly at their devices while texting.

My days in the hospital were spent in comfort. Not in my own comfort, but in my attempt to console very sick patients and those who loved them. That is gone from my life after fifty years of getting better at it.

There are no rounds to be made, no operations to perform, no clinics to manage, no films or charts to review, no advice to be offered, no explanations to be given to the families of the sick, no distraught residents and medical students to soothe, no meetings to attend, no papers to fill out, no "modules" to satisfy. Actually, I don't miss the modules. Now I have to find stuff to do. I read. I write. I think. I work in the yard and garden. I still teach a little. People I know and old patients call or email me for advice now and then. I volunteer at a variety of places. I can still run (well, sort of) so I do.

I spend a lot of time trying not to think about what I am un-becoming.

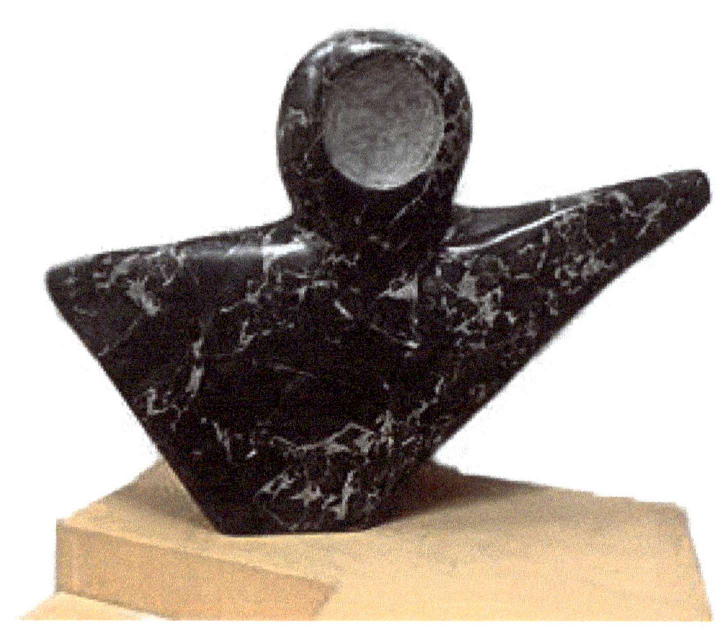

Reaching and Hope - marble by Kenneth Elconin, MD

A Fence or an Ambulance

By Monica L. Garrick Drago, MD
(Response to the original poem by Joseph Malins)

'Tis an interesting question I'm given to pose,
About being proactive or scooping up those
Whose curious nature has bettered their senses
And led to the question of putting up fences.

"Come to the crest!" all the risk-takers said.
They took every advantage, not using their heads,
To view the great scene just because they were able,
"We've no concern if that edge is not stable."

So, now, the dilemma presents to us all:
Should we pay for those willingly risking the fall?
They should have known better; we did, and we're fine.
Why help those who don't listen? Why use money of mine?

It's our duty, I say, to help others any way
Without fault being mentioned: white, black or gray.
They are victims, for sure, of their own mistake.
Yet, the care-taking role of society they make.

So the need for the ambulance is very clear,
For society's assistance should always be near.
But there lingers a role just as crucial as this:
That is, the *prevention* of victims in th'abyss.

If picking up pieces was all that we did,
The casualties mounting we never could rid.
Yes, to aid the fallen is expected indeed.
Acting to prevent harm, however, must supersede.

What, then, must we do to carry out our task?
We must advocate, educate *before* they ask.
We must steer them from dangers and unknown faux pas,
Collaborate, delegate-help make better laws.

We, as fence-builders, society shall see
Will save some the fall and spare many the bruised knee.
We must still tend the ambulance, bandages and all,
But the fence must be built and it needs to be tall!
Perhaps there's a compromise possible still
For those who insist that because of free will
The view from the crest should not shielded they be:
A pane in the fence, so that they may see.

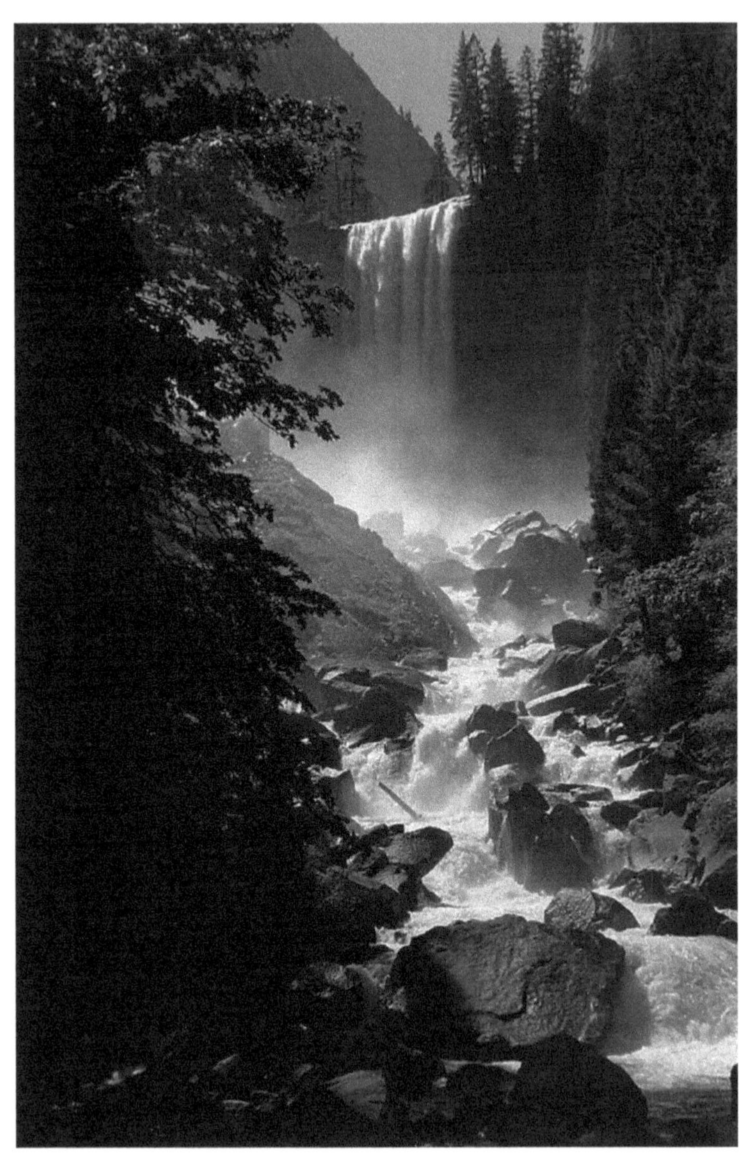

Mist Trail at Yosemite - photograph by Cynthia A. Point, MD

Why?

By Lois Freedman, MD

Why is human kindness so hard to teach?
Why does it seem the golden rule has been lost?
And how can we help those who follow in our footsteps,
rediscover the joys of medicine we experienced
in our beginnings in medicine?

As mentors can we help others
to pause and reflect,
to bring forth the possibility of the positive,
gentle, and healing aspects
of our chosen field?
I hope so.

Inspiration

By John M. Mazzullo, MD

One of the most exciting moments of my life was in 2008. A patient of mine endowed the "Mazzullo Lectureship in Primary Care." The patient wanted to be anonymous at first so this gift would not change our medical relationship. The lectureship's goal was to present topics of particular interest to me, focused mainly on issues of primary care that had always fascinated me during my career. The topics ranged from issues of HIV disease to the financial crises in medicine, to the development of hospice care. I tried to choose speakers who could speak to a diverse audience of clinicians and, most importantly, to former patients whom I especially wanted to attend. My patients were to be included because I had to retire suddenly without much warning due to a serious medical problem. Thus, I had no time to plan their future care or even to say good-bye.

I developed urothelial cancer in 2006. Ultimately, it spread through my entire urinary tract so by 2008, I lost both kidneys and started dialysis. In 2011, the cancer had spread to my lungs, so I needed surgery and more chemotherapy. During this time, I maintained my clinical work, but finally at this occurrence, it was the time to retire because the prognosis was grave.

In all, I did home hemodialysis for a total of seven years until 2015 when I was well enough to consider transplant. I was able to find a donor who had worked in the Kidney Division of my hospital where I started dialysis. When it came time for my transplant, my donor had already graduated from medical school and decided to give me one of his kidneys on May 12, 2015. After the transplant, I rejoined the faculty of the hospital and medical school in 2016 so that I could continue to teach students and residents, but I did not do any clinical care.

My patients all knew of my illness – how else could it be? I tried to continue to provide care to them even though I became a patient myself. The suddenness of my retirement prevented an individually structured termination of my care with them. I could not make specific referrals for each patient as I would have liked, depending on their disease and most importantly their particular circumstances. Sadly, they received a bureaucratic form letter informing them of my retirement with a choice of three newly hired doctors.

To somewhat make up for my sudden departure, this yearly lecture was more than a lecture but also a reunion for all of us to catch up and see each other in a nicer place with a wine-and-cheese reception before the lecture began.

For the tenth anniversary in 2018 of the lectureships, I tried to get Dr. Anthony Fauci to speak as he is one of my heroes, but he was too busy (even then!). By default, I became the speaker who tried to tell the personal story of the early days of the HIV epidemic. I attempted to weave the story of my becoming an HIV clinician, my coming out as a gay man, and my needing to become a patient dealing with my own deadly disease over a thirty-year period.

At the end, the audience, filled with my surviving patients and former colleagues, gave me a standing ovation that seemed like it would not stop. The fond memory of those smiling faces still gives me smiles and tears to this day.

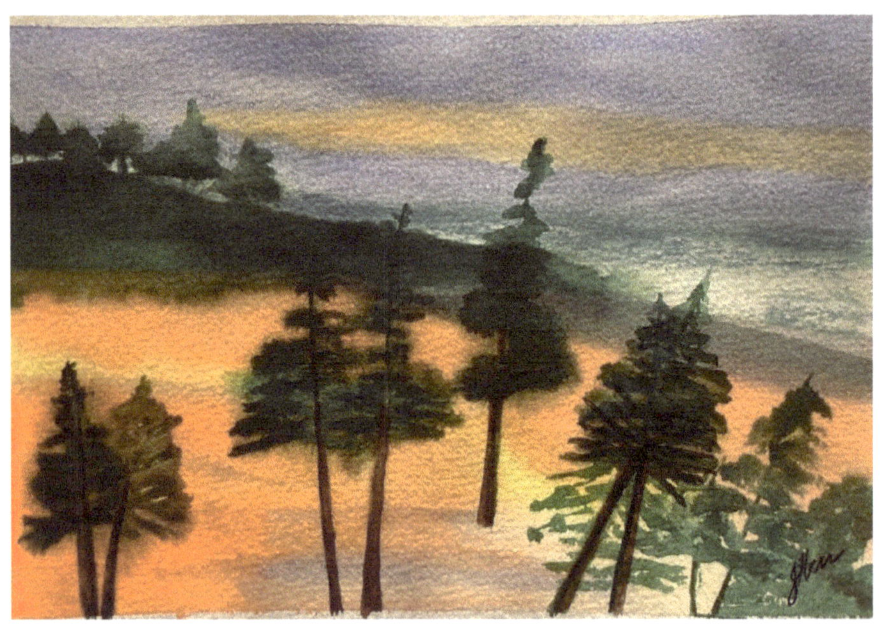

Trees - watercolor by Jan L. Herr, MD

The Pause That I Really Needed

By LoAn Nguyen, MD

In the early bright sun of a winter morning in February 2001, my husband J. and I had just finished a leisurely late breakfast and were comfortably settled in to read the weekend newspaper together. The brilliant sunlight was streaming in, promising a happy and peaceful morning. J. was sitting across the table; he had found an interesting article and decided to read it aloud to me. As he turned his neck, I noticed a marble-sized nodule in the location of his right thyroid gland. After he finished reading, I approached him to check out the nodule that had greatly distracted me. It was a firm, smooth, round mass palpable in the right thyroid bed. I felt a sharp jab in my heart as it slid under my fingers: A list of differential diagnoses quickly ran through my head. My calculation was that the worst probable scenario would be papillary or follicular thyroid cancer, which is very curable. I tried to appear calm and not terribly worried as I gently discussed with him what I had just found. I shared my thoughts of possibilities, including benign nodule to malignancy. We discussed the logistics of referrals and testing to be done.

Over the next few weeks, the evaluation process proceeded. First were blood tests and ultrasound, then a visit with an endocrinologist, who referred J. for biopsy of the nodule. I accompanied him for that procedure. I asked to take a peek at the slide that the pathologist prepared. With a glance through the microscope, I knew it was a malignancy. The exact type would depend on additional preparation and study.

A week later, we learned that the thyroid tumor was medullary thyroid cancer, a rare thyroid cancer, only one to two percent of all thyroid cancers in the U.S. His calcitonin, a tumor marker level, was quite high, in the five thousand range, though he was asymptomatic. I immediately searched the literature, trials, treatments and, of course, prognosis. Since it is an uncommon disease, prognostic information was not abundant, and what I found was not encouraging. Within a month J. underwent an eight-hour radical neck dissection followed by thirty-five days of grueling radiation therapy to both sides of his neck.

This turn of events was such a blow; I found myself terribly frightened. Our two daughters were only five and thirteen years old at the time. Ominous questions constantly raced through my head: will J. be there for birthdays, graduations, weddings? How would I manage without J. by my side, as he had been for the prior seventeen years?

Over the next several months I kept busy with work, J.'s treatments, and the children's routines. J.'s stoical attitude and coping skills were tremendously helpful as we tried to maintain a sense of normality for our daughters. But my anxiety and fear would surface during times of deep solitude, such as night hours when the house was quiet, with everyone peacefully in slumber. Day was not any kinder. What should have been a cheerful blue sky with birds chirping no longer brought peace and happy thoughts. Sunshine had fled, leaving only an ominous dark cloud over me.

My anxiety continued to escalate until I finally confronted myself. Where had my resilient self gone during this harsh chapter of life? The answer came from within: By Nature's fundamental design, life is transient and fleeting. I did not know what my "prognosis" was because

I did not have a serious diagnosis. Why did I continue to dwell on J.'s prognosis? I went back to one of Buddha's teachings that I learned long ago that was staying dormant within me: the desire to know the future, as well as the wish to keep what I have forever, was causing my suffering. From that moment of insight, pause and reflection, I learned to dissipate anticipation and desire for a certain future. I recalled many troubled times during the Viet Nam war, my years alone in the U.S. after the fall of Saigon, and how I had managed to survive. My recollections proved to be much better than what anti-anxiety medications could have offered in addressing the fundamental source of my unhappiness. I started to focus on what I had, rather than on what I might not have in the future; I remembered to treasure each and every life moment and not to dwell on when the moments might vanish. My tranquility began to be restored, sleepless nights gradually fading into shadows as I regained tranquility.

A great deal of human suffering derives from apprehension of the unknowable. I reminded myself and sometimes my patients that only people with a difficult diagnosis would ask for or be given a prognosis. The reality is none of us knows our prognosis at any given time. Learning to pause, reflect, and see beauty in many things which are presented to us is a worthy endeavor when we face life's challenge.

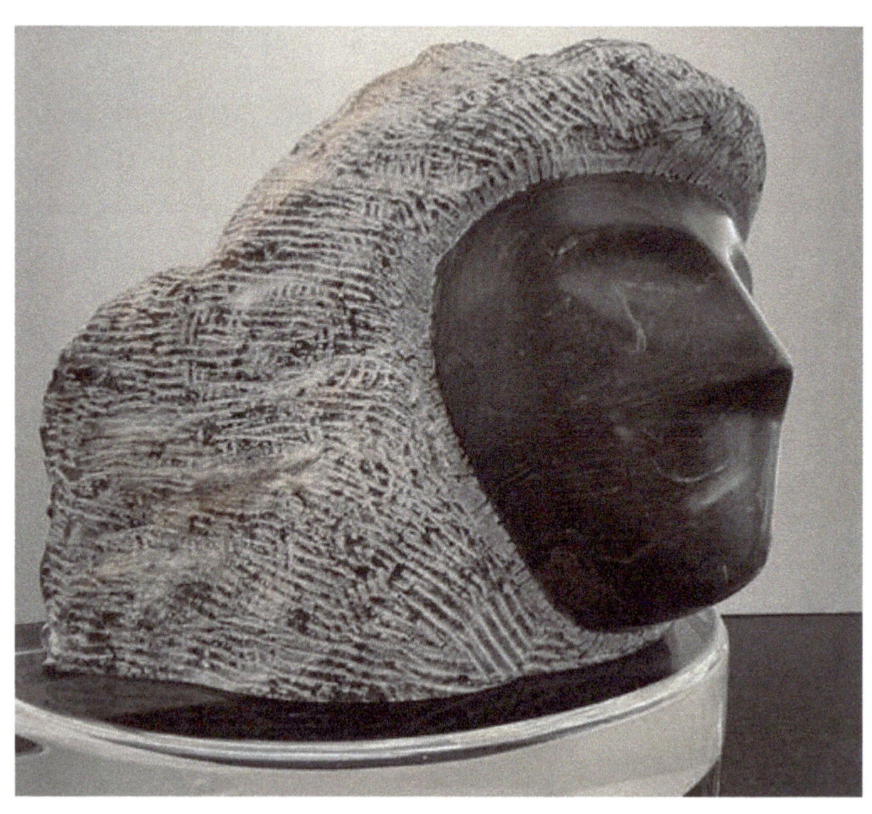

Sphinx #1 - marble by Kenneth Elconin, MD

How a Starbuck's Barista Renewed My Youth

By Scott Abramson, MD

I am seventy-four years old now.

When I was sixty-five, something happened that told me I was getting old.

Here is what it was:

As I walked out of my local Safeway grocery store, a pretty young woman smiled at me. My immediate reaction was not to smile back…but embarrassingly, I found myself glancing southward to make sure all was well in the "zip up" department.

It hit me then and there.

I was becoming an old person.

For the next month I wallowed in this muddy revelation.

I suspected I was clearly entering the early stages of geezerhood.

But alas, one month later, faith in my youthful, pre-geezer self-image was renewed. And amazingly enough, it was a barista working at Starbucks, who renewed it. I had ordered my usual cinnamon latte and three almond biscotti's. (I love those things) "You know," remarked the barista, "you can bake those biscotti's at home."

"Yeah," I mumbled, without much enthusiasm. "I guess so."

She gave me a long, lingering look (at least that's how I choose to recall the story now.)

"But you don't look like the kind of man," she smiled, "that spends his time baking in the kitchen."

Upon my sacred Medicare Advantage password, I swear to you, those were her exact words.

Meanwhile, I started thinking to myself (as I channeled my inner John Wayne.)

"You got that right, Missy.

I ride the range.

I corral them doggies.

I don't bake no biscotti."

Hell, I may be sixty-five, but now I'm feeling like a young buck inside!

So, what's the point?

It's the impact of a compliment:

It's the power of praise.

If, by simple kind words, a Starbuck's barista can make an old geezer like me feel good. Think about how each of us can make others feel uplifted and **renewed.**

Giddyap!

Epilogue

This collection reflects the time-travel experience of MAVEN Project physician volunteers. Our hope is that the book imparts both the uniqueness and the commonality of contributors' journeys. Like a kaleidoscope, each physician's life presents beautiful patterns and seemingly infinite colors that are connected in wonderful ways.

Acknowledgements

We thank the leadership of MAVEN Project for sponsoring this book and supporting the formation of the "Narrative and Humanity" writing group which created this collection.

We are very grateful to Dr. Jill Einstein, Senior Director of Physician Engagement for MAVEN Project. She is deeply committed to building a strong community of physician volunteers. This book is a testament to the value of opening space for connection and fellowship through stories and the impact it has had on our well-being.

We thank Linaise Lima, Physician Engagement Associate for MAVEN Project, for her commitment to this endeavor.

About the Authors & Artists

Scott Abramson, MD retired in 2020 after forty years of proudly practicing Neurology at the Kaiser Permanente Medical Group in Northern California. His passion is living the good life in retirement and his mission now is to spend whatever remains of his children's inheritance!

Grace D. Bandow, MD is a practicing dermatologist living in Wilton, CT, and a MAVEN Project volunteer. She is married, raising three stepchildren, loves to cook, exercise, and play the piano.

Susan Boiko, MD is a semiretired pediatric dermatologist who lives in San Diego and will be retiring from pediatric dermatology practice at UCSD soon. She is passionate about Community Outreach to underserved populations and about tasting every kind of chocolate.

Michael E. Day, MD lives and is licensed in Indiana. He still works part time in Family Medicine as well as doing volunteer mentoring and teaching. He enjoys traveling, hiking, golfing, and spending time with grandchildren and grand dogs.

Germaine L. Defendi, MD is a retired pediatrician who resides in South Pasadena, CA. She is currently a volunteer physician with MAVEN Project and is an author of Medscape articles. She is passionate about intellectual curiosity through creativity and exploration of the arts.

Henry W. Eisenberg, MD is a retired surgeon. His major activity, in addition to MAVEN Project, is the Cleveland Museum of Art where he volunteers in the library. He also enjoys golf when the weather permits.

Kenneth Elconin, MD is a retired orthopedic surgeon residing in Los Angeles. His current activities include being a Docent at the Getty Museum of Art, tennis, and three book clubs. For almost 40 years, he has been an active sculptor in a variety of media, primarily marble most recently.

Lois Freedman, MD is a retired general consultation liaison and geriatric psychiatrist currently living in Shaker Heights, Ohio. She is passionate about all living things.

Monica L. Garrick Drago, MD is a practicing behavioral medicine and addiction specialist in Pittsburgh, PA. She has three young adult children who make her proud every day. Dr. Drago is passionate about golf, piano and guitar, and loves to bake.

Jan L. Herr, MD is a semi-retired obstetrician gynecologist. She feels very fortunate to have had a rich and satisfying career at Kaiser Permanente Northern California after thirty-three years. Her leisure time is spent biking, hiking, painting, reading, and traveling (Covid permitting.)

Carrie A. Horwitch, MD is an outpatient internal medicine physician in Seattle, WA. She is also a certified laughter leader from World Laughter Tour. Her medical interests are HIV care, medical education, ethics, professionalism, and physician well-being. She also loves to travel, spend time with friends and family, Cajun, folk dancing, and reading.

David C. Hurwitz, MD is a retired rheumatologist living in Calabasas, California. He has participated in writing groups, and is active in community service, serving on the Calabasas Senior Center Steering Committee, and running the Senior Center Photography Club.

David P. Hurwitz, MD is a general internist residing in Melbourne, Florida. He currently works as a part time hospitalist. He is passionate about using health information technology to improve clinical outcomes and to reduce clinicians' work burden.

Vahe A. Keukjian, MD is a newly retired family physician still licensed in New York. He lives in Hudson Valley. He volunteers for several medical organizations as well as for Braver Angels, a non-profit organization dedicated to reconciliation across political and ideological divides. His personal quirks are too dull to catalogue.

Cynthia C. Leigh, MD is a retired endocrinologist from Neenah, WI, currently spending significant time in Minneapolis, MN to enjoy her new job as "Gramma". She trains with a master's swimming group in both locations and adapted to continuing harp lessons on Zoom.

Barbara Loeb, MD was raised in Chicago by a single mother, an artist and dancer, who instilled the importance of humanity and creativity into her children's upbringing. After medical school and residency, Dr. Loeb started an Internal Medicine practice, served as a physician leader and healthcare consultant. In 2021, she published a collection of poems accompanied by her mother's art, "How to Save a Life: Healing Power of Poetry."

John M Mazzullo, MD is a General Internal Medicine physician who retired after 35 years of general medicine practice with Tufts Medical Center. His special interests include all aspects of Internal Medicine especially, LGBTQ+ Health, HIV, Monkeypox, and COVID. He now volunteers for MAVEN Project and teaches medical student physical exam and diagnosis at Tufts, School of Medicine.

Peter M. McGough, MD is a retired Family Physician and Clinical Professor who previously served as the medical director for eighteen primary care clinics affiliated with UW (University of Washington) Medicine. He lives in Seattle with his wife and enjoys playing music and traveling.

Prasanna Menon, MD is a retired OBGYN who resides in San Francisco Bay Area. Currently she spends time volunteering at a local school, spending time with her grandchildren, learning composting, gardening, singing, and enhancing her understanding of spirituality.

LoAn Nguyen, MD was born in South Vietnam. She emigrated to the United States as a young refugee a few days before the Fall of Saigon in the spring of 1975. Dr. Nguyen retired after almost twenty-eight years of practice as a primary care internal medicine physician and leader. She resides in Vienna, Virginia and is married with two grown daughters and one grandchild.

Tom E. Norris, MD retired from the University of Washington after almost thirty years as an academic leader and family physician. He lives with his spouse, near his children and grandchildren, in NW Washington state. He is committed to "giving back" through volunteering.

John Orzano, MD is a retired family physician who resides in Manchester, NH. He practiced for over fifty years as a clinician, educator and researcher. He passionately spends his time with family, community, cooking, advocating for greater accessibility, the use of humor, and healing power of music.

Prasad Palakurthy, MD is a retired cardiologist and cardiac electro-physiologist, who currently lives in the East Bay Area, CA. He is a volunteer teacher of Yoga and Meditation in addition to being a volunteer physician.

Cynthia A. Point, MD is a retired Internist living in Northern California with her husband. She continues to ski, hike, and very importantly, spend outdoor time with her rescue dog. She enjoys being with her family and friends, and continues her photography. She notes that volunteering with MAVEN Project has been wonderful, allowing her to continue to use her knowledge and remain helpful.

Richard Rapport, MD is Clinical Professor Emeritus of Neurosurgery at the University of Washington School of Medicine and teaches at the Washington State University College of Medicine. He is licensed to practice in the State of Washington and lives in Seattle. He has been married to the writer of literary short fiction Valerie Trueblood for fifty years.

Jeanne Reisman, MD retired in 2018 after a thirty-four-year tenure in Primary Care and Health Education as part of the Kaiser Permanente Medical Group in Northern California. Dr. Reisman is also an artist, exploring different media and developing studio art practice. She and her husband love to garden, cook, and travel.

Craig Sadur, MD is a retired endocrinologist who resides in the San Francisco Bay Area and pursues various activities, including consultative and educational support for primary care clinicians through MAVEN Project. He is strongly motivated to stay current in adult endocrinology and help those clinicians with their patients regarding updated evidence-based and practical endocrine evaluation and management.

Charles E. Schwartz, MD is a retired academic internist and psychiatrist at Einstein Medical School, and lives in Manhattan. He works with NY State on medical care for the mentally ill; co-directs an addiction training program for residents; and is a founding member of the Association of Medicine and Psychiatry, dedicated to integrated med/psych care. He is a longtime MAVEN Project volunteer and mentor, and a writer.

Jill Silverman, MD is a retired internist and rheumatologist living in New York City. She is an amateur flutist who is involved with several chamber ensembles and is a volunteer with Sanctuary for Families, a non-profit organization helping women who have experienced domestic violence, and with the Weill Cornell Center for Human Rights and the Columbia Human Rights Initiative and Asylum Clinic.

Betsy Strong, MD was a primary care internist at Palo Alto Medical Foundation in Sunnyvale, CA for twenty years and retired in 2018. Her time is now divided between learning Spanish, volunteering as English Second Language (ESL) tutor, mentoring advanced practice providers with MAVEN Project, and enjoying time with her husband and family.

Bradley J. Winston, MD is a semi-retired Gastroenterologist and Hepatologist, former chief of GI/Hepatology Kaiser Permanente in the Mid-Atlantic States. He is passionate about health care, helping those who can't help themselves, human rights, health care reform, music, movies, singing, playing guitar, art collector on a budget, and now exploring the world of voiceovers.